YOGA

conditioning for

WEIGHT LOSS

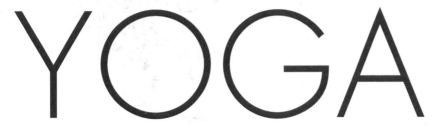

YOGA

conditioning for

WEIGHT
LOSS

Safe, natural methods

to help achieve

and maintain your

ideal weight

suzanne deason

RODALE

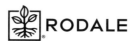

RODALE

WE **INSPIRE** AND **ENABLE** PEOPLE TO IMPROVE
THEIR LIVES AND THE WORLD AROUND THEM

Printed in the United States of America on acid-free ∞, recycled paper ♻

Editor: Margot Schupf

Cover and Interior Book Designer:
    Blue Cup Design, Inc., Wayne Wolf

Cover Photographer: David Safian

Interior Photographer: Ron Derhacopian

Layout Designer: Donna Bellis

Copy Editor: Nancy Rutman

Product Specialist: Brenda Miller

Indexer: Nanette Bendyna

Rodale Organic Living Books

Executive Editor: Margot Schupf

Art Director: Patricia Field

Content Assembly Manager:
    Robert V. Anderson Jr.

Copy Manager: Nancy N. Bailey

Editorial Assistant: Sara Sellar

We're always happy to hear from you. For questions or comments concerning the editorial content of this book, please write to:

Rodale Book Readers' Service

33 East Minor Street

Emmaus, PA 18098

Look for other Rodale books wherever books are sold. Or call us at (800) 848-4735.

For more information about Rodale Organic Living magazines and books, visit us at

www.rodale.com

Library of Congress Cataloging-in-Publication Data

Deason, Suzanne.
    Yoga conditioning for weight loss : safe, natural methods to help achieve and maintain your ideal weight / by Suzanne Deason.
        p.   cm.
        Includes index.
        ISBN 0–87596–912–7   (pbk. : alk. paper)
        1. Weight loss.   2. Yoga.   3. Reducing exercises.   I. Title.
        RM222.2 .D423 2003
        613.7—dc21   2002015742

Distributed in the book trade by St. Martin's Press

2   4   6   8   10   9   7   5   3   1   paperback

CONTENTS

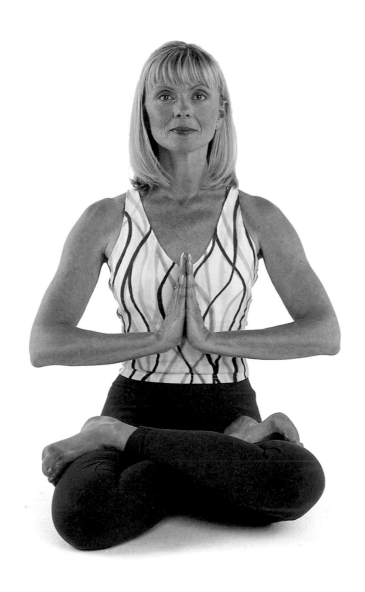

ACKNOWLEDGMENTS

Writing this book was an unexpected pleasure. From the very start, I had the good fortune to be supported by a talented team of people who were all "on the same page." During the process, the pieces just seemed to fall into place—something that can happen only as a result of hard work and communication. I want to say thanks to everyone who showed up to do their job so professionally and with such dedication in the interest of the greater good.

I'd like to thank Kerry Eielson for hours of fun and inspiring transcontinental phone conversations, from which she skillfully took my thoughts and experiences and put them down on paper in just the right way.

I would like to recognize the support and cooperation of the people at Gaiam, especially Lynn Powers, who believed in the importance of this project, and Howard Ronder, who gave valuable creative input. And a special thanks to Andrea Lesky, who, in the 11th hour, showed up with creativity and tenacity and took this book across the finish line.

I'm very grateful to have worked with the people at Rodale: Nancy Bailey, Patricia Field, Nancy Rutman, and particularly Margot Schupf, my editor, whose seamless editing, knowledge of yoga, and faith in the book made the work of putting it together feel effortless. Thanks also to designer Wayne Wolf and Los Angeles–based photographer Ron Derhacopian.

Without the success of the *Yoga Conditioning for Weight Loss* video, this book may not have been possible. Thanks to Marne Shapiro, Merrily Milmoe, and Veronica De Martini, who cheerfully practiced their parts and showed us that yoga *is* for everybody.

The nutrition information in Chapter 3 was greatly informed by conversations with James Rouse, N.D., director of coordinated care for the Phoenix Center of Health Excellence in Denver, Colorado. Dr. Rouse is a naturopathic physician and is also the wellness anchorperson for *Fit Kitchen*, on KUSA, NBC's Denver affiliate.

I would like to acknowledge Patricia Walden, a woman who exemplifies the integrity that yoga teaches. Thank you for inspiring me and for raising the bar for all of us.

To my yoga teacher, Judith Lasater: My years with you come through in every class I teach, and your wit and wisdom still touch my heart and make me smile.

Finally, special thanks to all of my students. Your trust, enthusiasm, and willingness to share your time and your lives with me are precious gifts.

Namaste.

INTRODUCTION

Forget, for just a moment, your desire to shed pounds and drop clothing sizes.

Stop counting.

Let go of feeling fat.

Take a few minutes to imagine life without the pressure to be anything other than yourself. Envision that self as the healthy, fit, balanced person you were born to be. Feel the freedom of being comfortable with who you are.

You may be picking up this book as part of a lifelong struggle against fat and calories, a battle waged on the geography of your own body. It's time to disengage from that struggle. The first step will be to let go of impossible expectations realized via unhealthy means and pay attention to your true self. Yoga can help you accomplish this.

Yoga leaves people with awakened senses, a feeling of fulfillment, and simplified, newly aligned priorities. Yoga clears mental clutter and disguise and brings forth the authenticity of the soul. It helps people to lead genuine lives guided by realistic desires and a grounded focus on health and well-being. It helps us establish a balanced relationship with ourselves and the natural world.

Ultimately, a yoga practice can help you to fulfill your potential on every level. The result will be far more lasting and valuable than any quick-fix weight loss program: a familiarity and self-awareness—emotionally, physically, mentally, and spiritually—that can put your body and your life back in perspective. With regular practice, your mind, body, and spirit will be guided toward optimum health; your thoughts will be clearer, your actions more genuine, and your body stronger, leaner, and more efficient.

How does it work? If we are serious about making lasting changes in our lives, we must have all aspects of ourselves moving toward the desired result. The concentration on postures and breathing that yoga develops shifts our focus away from external distractions and guides us inside ourselves where our thought and emotions determine our external behavior and actions. Yoga serves as a tool to unite and integrate our wholeness. It gently reintroduces us to ourselves. It relieves us of petty concerns and redirects our energy to the present moment, where we have the power of choice.

The key to making your yoga practice complete will be to take this heightened knowledge of yourself and use it to make a realistic connection to the healthy life that you desire and to the world. One very important tenet of yoga is to honor all life. By teaching us to understand ourselves and to feel compassion for ourselves, yoga teaches empathy. The practices in this book will strengthen your foundation so that you can extend your connectedness to all living things.

Self-knowledge will improve your relationships and ability to communicate. Self-worth will help you find a release from fear and unhealthy attachments. Self-respect and a conscious approach to all you do will change your attitude about health and lifestyle.

We have been given this beautiful life, one that many of us drag around like a cumbersome suitcase. Yoga will help awaken a deeper sense of who you are, a desire to be your absolute best, and a kind of reverence for the vehicle you use to move through life from birth to death. If you practice with patience, commitment, and consistency, this respect for your body and an increased consciousness about the decisions you make (not to mention the strengthening, toning, and metabolism-boosting benefits of yoga as a physical exercise) will lead you to a more balanced approach to food, a more vital body, and a balanced mind.

Use yoga to lighten the burdens. It's an honor and a privilege to take care of the bodies we've been given and to be able to extend that gift to others—to our children, our families, and our communities. You've been given something beautiful. It's time to enjoy it!

Part One: The Mind-Body Connection

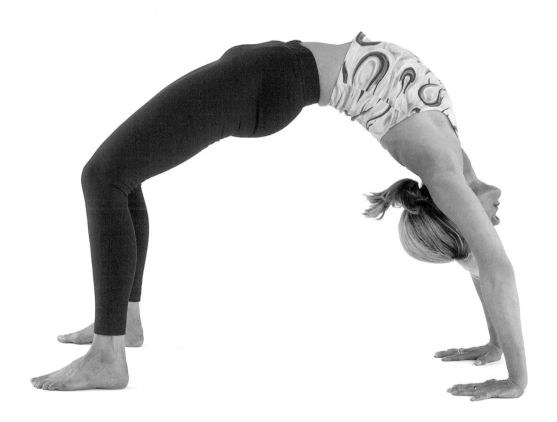

[1]

WHY YOGA FOR WEIGHT LOSS?

While the title of this book is *Yoga Conditioning for Weight Loss,* it may surprise you to learn that weight loss is not entirely the point. Yoga is certainly a means to that end, but not exactly in the way one would expect. Yoga helps you to develop a leaner, more supple body not by emphasizing a restricted food intake and targeted muscle-building but by nurturing an attitude adjustment that paves the way for long-term change. Yoga establishes physical and mental poise in a natural, gradual, lasting, and organic way.

Typical weight loss programs address the symptom (excess fat) and ignore the cause, which is essentially an imbalance caused by or manifested as any range of emotional problems, bad habits, and poor nutrition. Through a sustained yoga practice, your body will change, your health and metabolism will improve, your peace of mind and self-discipline will return. If you opened this book strictly with the desire to slim down, you've come to the right place, but be prepared to experience wonderful mental, emotional, and spiritual side effects!

Diets Don't Work

The first reason to turn to yoga is simple: Diets—at least the type of diets most people follow—don't work. The ancient Greek word *diaita* meant "manner of living." Diets in our society are usually defined as "food-deprivation regimens that promote temporary thinness." What a difference!

Think of your "diet" in the ancient Greek way: Your diet is your way of life. You can't separate your behavior with food from your relationship with the rest of the world. If you are starving yourself, or cheating or being dishonest with yourself in terms of food, chances are you are doing it elsewhere. On the other hand, if you have an exciting, nurturing, and enthusiastically healthy way with food, that openness and generosity of spirit will extend to the rest of your life.

You may have tried traditional diets and all they engender: dashed expectations and frustration, poor eating habits, mean cravings, chronic hunger, low energy, caloric restrictions, weight fluctuation, confused metabolism, and a menu that leaves a great deal to be desired.

Food-restriction and food-substitution diets don't work over the long run because they are not intended for long-term weight loss. The diet industry is big business. It spends $100 billion a year on products and marketing. Every year, about 92 percent of people buying those products are return customers. So 9 out of 10 diets fail! If diets really worked, their creators would go out of business. Most diet companies simply do not have your best interests in mind. They do very little to encourage the permanent lifestyle changes necessary to achieve a long-term goal. And diets don't address the emotional issues of weight gain.

We all know the formula for losing weight: Burn more calories than you consume. If it's so easy, why are 60 percent of Americans overweight? The reason is that, although weight gain has something to do with how much and what we eat, it often has more to do with *why* we eat, which varies considerably from person to person.

If you're eating to compensate for grief, dieting won't help you deal with your loss. If you snack to calm your nerves, cutting calories won't help you release stress. If you crave the wrong foods because of chemical imbalances, an appetite suppressant won't recalibrate your system. If you indulge in bad habits with the excuse that your job is too demanding and you simply don't have time to maintain a more balanced lifestyle, a frozen low-fat meal won't help you take responsibility for your health and well-being.

Many bad habits are emotionally driven; their catalyst may be a single act of self-neglect that spirals into a breakdown in the system. You can't stop the downward spiral until you have located the root of self-neglect. By teaching you to turn your focus inward, yoga works on an emotional level to put you in touch with your feelings and to strengthen a nurturing relationship with yourself. By increasing your awareness of your body and the way we move through life, yoga can help you recognize how and why you aren't taking better care of yourself. It can help you identify your overeating triggers and determine whether they are chemical, habitual, or emotional.

Yoga also works on a biological level to offset the reactions that are set in motion when you eat unhealthy foods, or foods that may be right for others but wrong for you. These foods cause hormonal reactions that can lead not only to obesity and disease but also to depression, a common trigger for bingeing. Depression is an overeating trigger that actually has a foundation in nutrition and body chemistry as well as in life experience or brain chemistry. Eating "wrong" foods tips off a reaction that often simultaneously makes us crave more of the same and drives us deeper into depression.

By tracking how your body and feelings relate to food, you can find the keys to maintaining equilibrium—both emotional and biological. That's something most diets just won't do. Diets are often about limiting your experience. Yoga is about celebrating the experience of life. Which would you find easier to commit to?

Exercise Isn't Enough

Cardiovascular exercises, such as jogging and aerobics, are very effective ways of burning calories fast and reducing stress temporarily. When practiced mindfully and sensibly, they can be a great complement to a healthy regimen.

Unfortunately, most people don't approach cardiovascular exercise programs from a holistic perspective. Our bodies work in many ways; we naturally seek and need diversity of movement. Many kinds of exercise don't address or take advantage of the whole body, and when people fall into exercise ruts, they don't use their bodies in all their capacities and they don't make the mind-body connection so essential to mental and physical health.

Think about it: A lot of people do the same single exercise for years on end, working one set of muscles in exactly the same way for the same amount of time. Some of the muscles in our very complex body never get any of the benefits of increased circulation, strengthening, and lengthening. When our intention is focused either on burning the maximum number of calories in a half-hour or on repeatedly contracting and relaxing one muscle, such as the hamstrings, we end up with poor alignment, muscular imbalances, and potentially, repetitive stress injury.

Such modes of exercise are also not at all appropriate for people who aren't already physically fit. Take your average American, for example—someone who drives instead of walking, takes the elevator instead of the stairs, sits for hours in front of the TV (using the remote instead of getting up to change the channel), and slouches behind a desk for at least eight hours a day! Let's call this "someone" Joe. Joe wakes up one day after seeing his fit cousin Ronnie and looks in the mirror. Joe is tired of feeling heavy and tired, sick of being flaccid and unfit. So, in a burst of enthusiasm, Joe hits the streets. He plans to jog 2 miles every other day and do 30 situps every morning to drop 10 pounds by June 1, just as that fitness magazine suggested. Chances are he'll be so sore after one day, he may feel as if he'll never be able to move again, let alone run.

Jogging alone, as one example, does very little to change unhealthy patterns that are so often behind weight gain. You may successfully achieve a fitter-looking frame after a few weeks of jogging, but as soon as you get busy, hurt yourself, or go on vacation, you'll put the weight right back on, because you still have the same eating habits and mental reflexes.

The same goes for the gym. Gym workouts don't typically strengthen the mind-body connection. Gym culture is often a critical and competitive environment, whether it's because you have to jockey for position in line at a treadmill or because you have to follow the barking commands of a harsh trainer. Just getting to the gym can be a hassle on top of other hassles. When you can't get there, you feel you've fallen behind; all it takes to get off track is one busy week. You get busy, you can't get to the gym, you get derailed, you gain weight and become discouraged.

The key to a healthy lifestyle lies with your intention. Yoga works on your intention. It is a practice you can do at home or take with you anywhere—a frame of mind you can tap into all day to stay balanced and focused. Do any exercise you want, but do it mindfully. Pay attention to your limits. Start slowly and become conscious of your body.

But use your body whenever you can. Our bodies love to move. Discover your versatility. Dancing, bicycling, swimming, Pilates, martial arts, and other forms of exercise are great complements to a fit lifestyle, but they should be incorporated with stretching and strengthening exercises to reduce the risk of injury and breathing exercises to encourage the mind-body connection and its emphasis on holistic health. Flex your perspective.

YOGA SUTRA 2:55...
*From this comes supreme
mastery of the senses.*

What Is Yoga?

Yoga is a physical and spiritual practice developed in India more than 5,000 years ago. It was designed to prepare the body for meditation by enabling a person to remain seated for long periods and to "open" the body so that energy could flow freely during meditation. The word *yoga* may be translated literally as "yoking," from the Sanskrit *yunatki* ("he yokes"), and implies both integration between mind and body and, on a larger level, peace between self and world.

The most commonly known yoga in the West is called hatha yoga. Hatha means the integration of sun and moon, which refers to the integration of mind and body that is experienced in yoga practice. Hatha yoga is practiced by placing the body in different postures called *asanas.* Yoga *asanas* involve detailed, precise movement; the mind is active in the performance of every *asana* in order to improve discipline and create awareness, which also helps to maintain the posture.

The word *asana* means "ease" in Sanskrit. The mind and body reach a state of relaxation and ease that helps stimulate the circulation of *prana,* or life force. This state of being produces a feeling of wholeness, integration, and purpose, which extend to a feeling of spiritual connection to all life. A properly executed *asana* creates a balance between exertion and surrender, between movement and stillness. This is the optimal state of balance for human life to exist.

Mind-Body Fitness Is the Answer

An authentic desire to lead a healthy lifestyle exists within everyone. But many of us have been out of touch with our bodies and out of balance for so long, we don't even know we feel bad. If we do, we can't quite make out where to begin to feel better. The answer is, start simply, start from the core, and go for a change that will impact your life on every level.

The mind-body connection we find through yoga is the missing link to making a lasting change to a healthy lifestyle. It all starts with paying attention to how you feel. By concentrating the mind on the body and bringing its focus inward, away from the complex web of artificial obligations we wrap ourselves in, yoga brings the mind into a relationship with the body that encourages and supports striving for wellness and good health. It's hard not to do what's best for our health when we go through our day mindfully and consciously.

When your mind and body work in tandem, you are an active participant in everything you do. Life is more fulfilling. Instead of being just a body walking down the street, sitting in front of a television, munching on a bowl of popcorn, or standing in line at the bank, instead of being one of those people who pretends to be listening while the mind darts here and there, you will be a person with a purpose. You will be awake and engaged in your activities.

Recognize the beauty of your life. Accept the privilege to respect that body, take care of it, and use it to the best of its ability. No matter what you think about yourself on your worst day, you are blessed with this life. Make the most of every moment.

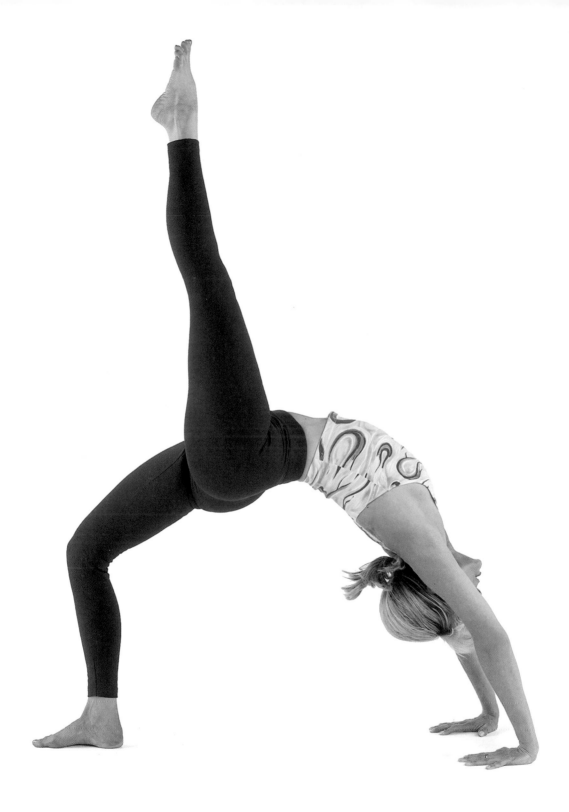

Willpower versus Inner Strength

The success of any commercial weight loss program usually depends on attachment to a goal. Goals often quickly lead to a fixation on something external, be it the number of calories or fat grams consumed in a day or pounds lost on a scale. Often our commitments to that program don't come easily because that goal is abstract and has nothing to do with who we are or how we really feel. Like New Year's resolutions, most goals are impersonal and unrealistic. (Can anyone really change overnight?) Goals create expectations without any regard for the individual or the self. And too often, goals are based on who we think we should be rather than who we are authentically.

The setting of unrealistic goals—and the all-but-guaranteed failure to attain those goals—is the perfect excuse to drop out before you've even hit your stride.

How many times have you purposely set a goal artificially high to motivate yourself to get at least mostly there? This is dishonest: It's not an attempt to be your best. Never promise yourself something that you don't intend to produce. Your subconscious can't take a joke, and you'll end up feeling like a failure on a very profound level. The negative cycle of self-fulfilled prophecies will begin, even if your desire to attain the goal was originally sincere.

Goals require willpower. Willpower is like the carrot that keeps the carriage horse going: Its pursuit is sheer drudgery. When you lose sight of the carrot due to fatigue or distraction, your pursuit of the goal is easily forgotten. All the willpower in the world does nothing to change the foundation of unhealthy patterns. Willpower is not grounded in authentic desire; it does not come from within; it is not genuine. How can you expect it to last?

Goals may get away from you, but a spiritually rooted sense of purpose will stay with you forever. You can take it anywhere and adapt it to your life at any moment. A spiritually rooted sense of purpose is individual and comes from a place of inner strength. You can't lose track of it.

The mind-body connection builds the inner strength that takes the place of willpower.

Remember, any improvement is a process. You can't change overnight. If you do let your yoga program lapse for a week or two, it's not likely to cause a mudslide of unhealthy routines. Yoga works on a holistic level and extends to all that you do. Once developed, inner strength takes a long time to lose. You are committed to a balanced life. You are not a quitter. You are simply a very busy person. What's one week? It's pretty insignificant in the big picture. This is your life we're talking about.

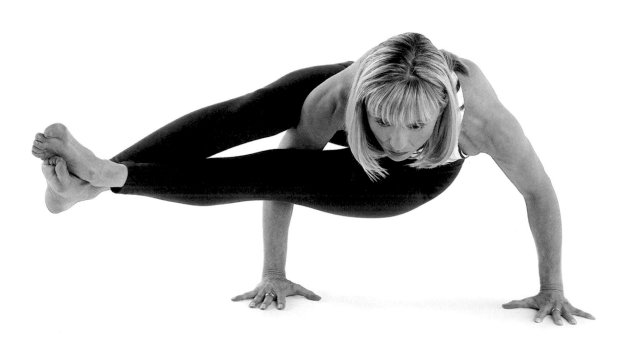

[2]

FINDING BALANCE

If leading a balanced life were entirely up to us, we wouldn't have to work so hard at it. Authenticity and balance exist within all of us—we are born with both. It shouldn't require such a conscious effort to be in touch with ourselves and live authentically, but it does. The pull of popular culture is very powerful, and we want to be a part of it all. But most aspects of modern life actually work against our natural rhythms. How do we reconcile simple, pure inner ideals with a world that, on the surface at least, seems to reserve so little regard or time for them?

It's always best to know what you're up against. Maybe you won't be so hard on yourself after you read this.

The Challenges of Modern Life

Our roles in society are becoming ever more multifaceted. With freedom of choice come many options, some of which are just too hard to turn down. We want it all, and that takes money. Money comes from hard work. Americans put in more hours per week than workers in any other country in the world, even Japan; it's been estimated that the average American works a 60-hour week.

On top of this, we have other roles with our families, social lives, hobbies, and indulgences. Each of us wants to be a perfect parent, spouse, daughter, or son, as well as a successful professional. We want to be up on the latest television show, movie, book, magazine article, and computer program; or we want to help our kids compete with the latest GameBoy, cool birthday party, or sneakers.

No one likes to be left behind. So we plug in and play the game, and we learn to do so at an early age. One town in New Jersey actually had to get the school board, sports coaches, and leaders of after-school activities together with parents and children to come up with one night a week when families could spend an evening together!

The fact is, our desire to interact with people often puts us in the company of a community that has largely unhealthy routines. We do too much and get stressed out. Medical science has shown us how detrimental stress is to our health, and that stress has become an inherent product of contemporary life. To save time, we all eat poorly, exercise less, and lose sleep. Research has shown that if allowed to live by natural rhythms, a human being would sleep for up to 15 hours. How many hours do you sleep?

In our effort to keep up and play a part, we forget ourselves. Our oversaturated minds become disconnected from our bodies, our actions become detached from our intentions, and we lose our center. We lose our rhythm and fall apart.

Expectations

Living according to others' expectations is a problem of inauthenticity to which we are all prone to some degree. The problem comes in when we follow any path for years without really thinking about whether we want to. Then we wake up one morning and realize how shallow we are, how uninterested in our own lives we have become.

The temptation here is to say, "But I'm not shallow, my life is." The point is, if you are living authentically, you are not separate from your life. You are reflected in your choices. If you are not invested in the things you choose, you simply cannot reach your potential and will not make the most of all you've been given. When you're doing something you don't really want to do, you'll eventually treat it with indifference. If you neglect yourself, you will ultimately neglect your job, friends, and family.

Where is your focus? For life to be authentic, and for your relationship to the world and to other people to be healthy and kind, your focus must start with yourself. When it does, your attention to other details in life will become genuine. Just as things that are right for others aren't necessarily right for you, things that are not right for you might be exactly what someone else is looking for. Leave the "wrong" life for someone who would be thrilled to have it. Look at who you really are. Learn how to express yourself best and you will go through life gracefully.

Negativity

With all the busyness and outward focus, it's easy to fall out of touch with emotions. Our experience becomes muted. Many of us exist nervously in such an emotional void: falling through space waiting to latch on to the first big feeling that comes along. If we have neglected ourselves, that emotion is often an angry one.

Anger and other negative emotions, such as jealousy and sadness, make us feel alive and give us a skewed sense of purpose. So, in a life that leaves us feeling disconnected from ourselves, we tend to experience overblown emotions. The extremes of this are physical abuse, road rage, workplace shootings, and even suicide. On a less horrific level, we are simply addicted to problems. We unintentionally get all worked up over life's insignificant complications. It's often called being "beside yourself." It's easy to let ourselves get carried away with negative missions.

Many people have never connected to the space of tranquility inside themselves. Instead of feeling nothing all day and then indulging in a wave of anxiety or insecurity, make it a part of your off-the-mat yoga practice to *feel* in everything you do. It doesn't have to be deep. It doesn't have to move mountains. But if you tap into the well of feeling inside you, that source of calm, you will be anchored and will feel more.

Escapes

No wonder we need escapes! But because we can't hightail it to a beach in Hawaii or Tahiti every time we get oversaturated, we space out.

Our culture finds it strange to sit and do nothing. Instead, we space out with our "poison" of choice: Smokers take a break from work and stare into the distance with their cigarettes; compulsive eaters relax at the end of a day with bowls of popcorn or ice cream; drinkers watch the soothing tonic of their alcohol drain from a glass; clotheshorses take in a few outfits on a Saturday-afternoon spree. Our means of escape seem always to be connected to action, which becomes habit, unconscious and unhealthy, and often a waste of time and energy. These are external stimulants that take the focus outside.

Be present in your enjoyment of everything you do. Nourish your mind, body, and spirit every day. You'll find it much more restorative than the television.

Detachment

Perhaps you looked out at life long ago and decided you'd sit this one out. You decided to stop punishing yourself, to stop trying to be someone else, and to stop trying to get others to relate to you. You got stuck in your escape. Chances are you are not making the most of all you've been given; you've stopped learning and exploring.

The good news is, if you are already detached, it may be easier for you to turn in and make the mind-body connection than it will be for others; you've already unhooked yourself from social expectations and other seductions of a modern life. Many people who have withdrawn just don't know the next step. All you have to do is find the desire—and that may not be easy.

Spirituality is about becoming the best one can possibly be. It's about expressing the best of what one has been given. You've been given legs; use them to walk. You've been given eyes; use them to see for those who can't. Recognize and use the blessings expressed in your body. To heal, you have to have this kind of spiritual connection. You have to believe in the good in yourself and the good in the world and set up a constant, lively exchange from one to the other. Become one with your body and one with your life. There's nothing more spiritual than that. This is about finding your humanity, reaching deep down, and coming out with your personal best to share it with the world. Yoga will be your guide to that discovery. It will help give you the confidence and the strength to face your self and share it with the world again.

YOGA SUTRA 2:33...
When negative feelings restrict us,
the opposite should be cultivated.

Genuine Priorities

Perhaps the greatest obstacle people think they face with regard to fitness is time, or the lack of it. You may be wondering how you'll ever get through this book, let alone do the postures. You're probably thinking, "Yeah, this is a great idea and I know it would work, but how will I fit it in?"

The first step will be to step out of our culture's paradigm of time, the *chronos* paradigm. Stop thinking about time as a sequence of seconds, equal in value and finite in quantity, that you must divide up and assign to an endless number of activities and responsibilities. Stop thinking of time as something to try to control. We can't determine the amount of time we have in a day, or in a life.

Forget about time management—that's not what this is about. It's about getting to what's essential. Think of time in terms of the quality of each moment. This is the definition of the *kairos* paradigm, still existent in certain cultures. View time with the interest of getting the most quality out of every moment, not fitting the most activities into each minute. This is not about finding time to practice yoga. This process is about getting in touch with your consciousness and your authentic self and consequently making better decisions about how to spend the time you already have.

Don't let your personality splinter. Pull back and gather all of your abilities and qualities at once. Have a holistic way of moving through each day. Be thoughtful in line at the grocery store, stretch at your desk at work, give yourself time to engage in friendly and interesting conversations with people over lunch. This may sound simple, but it is just too difficult to go about life any other way. Make your time rich. Try it—even if just for one week. You'll find it comes more naturally and instinctively than dividing each area of your life and personality into regiments housed in distinct boxes.

The clarity of mind instilled by yoga leads to an organic shift in priorities. It doesn't happen overnight, but you will discover more time in your schedule as certain commitments and obligations become less important and fall away from your day.

You might be thinking, "Wait, I want things to change, I want my body to change, but I want my life to stay the same!" Remember: Nothing will be taken away from you. If certain things fall away from your life, it will be when and because you don't want them anymore.

If you don't understand this concept, wait until you've had several months of consistent yoga practice. Once your senses awaken, you'll seek real experiences in the present; you'll choose to feel alive all the time. Instead of watching two hours of random television or flipping through a magazine every day to zone out, you may choose to garden, go for a walk, talk to friends and family, write letters, keep a journal. Maybe you'll rediscover a love of drawing and painting. The point is, you will seek out activities that fulfill your authenticity and deepen your connection with yourself and the world.

When you are focused, you will be more productive; when you feel centered and calm, you will find efficient solutions. *Do* less and *be* more. You'll be amazed at how much time you will have.

YOGA SUTRA 2:43...
From contentment, unsurpassed happiness is gained.

Making Choices

The real challenge with yoga is not only to find our place of inner strength on the mat but to be able to take that strength off the mat and maintain it in the face of all this distraction, mad consumption, and external stimulation. We clearly need to rethink, reprioritize, and simplify what is important. We do choose how we live our lives.

Yoga helps us do that. In the yoga practice, as the body moves through the poses, the mind is focused on breath, fluidity of movement, and alignment. It's simply not an option to think about other things for any long period of time. As you focus the mind on the breath, you link your attention and awareness to the internal self and establish an anchor to that place. This is where you begin to discover authenticity.

At the same time, stretching and contracting the muscles opens the body and improves circulation; it brings your focus to the body, part by part, and wakes it up. Yoga literally revives you physically, mentally, and spiritually. It is here that you begin to develop a relationship with yourself that is based on peace. Through the practice, you peel through physical and emotional layers of a shell you've developed over the course of your life. Each slight, each disappointment becomes a layer you use to protect your inner self. During practice and after practice, you begin to nurture that self and become familiar with it. You make it stronger. At some point, you tap into the source of peace and centeredness even when you're off the mat. The layers of disguise and armor become less necessary and eventually will be left by the wayside. Your strong inner self will be the self you put out to the world.

With this foundation, you will feel grounded and able to sit peacefully. You will move through your day with grace and poise—internal and external. Distractions won't be compelling to you anymore. You'll be awake. You'll feel alive. You won't need confirmation that you exist. You won't have to be defined by society in order to feel like you are a part of it.

At the same time, your ability to empathize will come naturally and take the place of a lot of negative reactions. You won't be as quick to attach yourself to insecure and vengeful feelings. When you realize what makes you act the way you do, you will understand other people's motivations and recognize their fears and weaknesses. We all act on personal impulses that have little to do with others. You'll look at a person who's just been nasty and instead of getting hurt or angry, you will feel for him or her. And you will forgive. You'll just say, "That person sure must be having a bad day." Life is difficult. You learn compassion as you exercise clarity.

The peace you find with yoga will serve as a constant reminder that you are alive and that you have a purpose: to reconnect with that spiritual life force, to redefine, reinvent, and redirect that thing inside that pushes you toward authenticity. It's a process of self-realization.

Change on Many Levels

On a **physical level,** the poses, breathing, and meditation that make up the yoga practice will, when combined and consistently practiced over time, work to lengthen and tone your muscles, burn fat, improve your posture, boost your metabolism and all bodily functions, calm your nervous system, lower your heart rate, and break the chain of chemical reactions in the body caused by stress and improper nutrition.

On an **emotional level,** yoga's postures and breathing techniques will increase your self-confidence, enable you to gain control over what were once involuntary emotional reactions, and cultivate a sense of calm. Learning to focus on the present will allow you to loosen attachments to anxiety, fear, and expectations and neutralize some overeating triggers.

Eventually, through the process of doing yoga, you will experience a shift in **perceptions.** You'll become centered and feel clearer about what you need. You'll be invigorated by a new sense of purpose. You will experience an awakened feeling of control over your life, a desire to take responsibility, and a deeper sense of investment in all that you do.

In terms of lifestyle, this stronger foundation will provide guidance in day-to-day decisions, including your **eating patterns.** You will be more aware of the food you put in your mouth and how it makes you feel. Your dietary choices and behavior will be shifted more toward health and well-being than cravings and convenience.

But before I talk specifically about nutritional strategy and the postures, I need to address the **attitude** adjustment you must make in order to successfully incorporate this practice into your life. Change is not going to happen by magic. It will not happen out of the blue, or as a result of wishing for it—though sincere desire is an essential starting point. If you want change in your life, *you* have to change the way you live. You must consciously nurture the desire to attain balance in your life, make that longing clear to the world, and then purposefully make the changes necessary to reach that place of equilibrium. It's up to you to take the reins.

YOGA SUTRA 1:29...
*Then the mind will turn inward
and the obstacles that stand in the way
of progress will disappear.*

3 Principles of Yoga

Yogic scholars believe that the mind and body are one, and that mental or physical distress can create illness. They recognize the potential of a vicious cycle of imbalance from one to the other. When our bodies are stagnant, so are our minds. When our minds are clouded, we forget to seek the pleasure of movement.

When we are able to manage our minds and thoughts, we become accountable for our behavior and quality of life and strive to improve both. Three of the most important principles of yoga: (1) discipline, of both body and mind; (2) clarity; and (3) freedom, meaning the ability to let go of unhealthy attachments. Attainment of all three objectives leads to a state of balance or serenity, known as *samadhi*. The yoga postures *(asanas)* and focused breathing *(pranayama)* restore the mind to simplicity and peace and free it from confusion and distractions, bringing the practitioner to a place of heightened awareness, understanding, and vision.

Discipline

The mind is like a monkey, swinging from thought to thought to thought. Without the focus that comes from meditation and yoga, getting hold of our thoughts can be just as difficult as it would be to catch that monkey with bare hands. As a result, many of us go through life only half aware of what we're doing, while the rest of our consciousness is awash with things that are ultimately irrelevant to our lives and utterly beyond our control.

In yogic thought, there are five states of mind, from the least disciplined to the highest, most focused and liberated state. These five characterizations are (1) dull and lethargic, (2) distracted, (3) scattered, (4) focused, and (5) disciplined.

See if you recognize yourself in any of these thought patterns and behaviors:

The **dull and lethargic mind** is stagnant and frustrated. Its symptoms include depression, withdrawal, disappointment, and disillusionment—symptoms that are exacerbated by compulsive eating and substance abuse. (People with borderline eating disorders usually fall into this category.)

The **distracted mind** is active but disoriented; feelings and thoughts dart and zip around in the brain without function or foundation.

The **scattered mind** develops perceptions but lacks direction; it is unanchored and breeds doubt, fear, and insecurity.

The **focused mind** is organized and aware, free of complications and complexes. People with focused minds live in the present; they don't let their choices be driven by the question "What if?"

Finally, the most elevated state is that of the **disciplined mind:** serene, steady, and composed. This state is one of absolute freedom, focus, and vision.

The yoga postures *(asanas)* themselves will work to help you discipline your mind. And to accompany them, there are other exercises that work to much the same effect. One of them is meditation—a technique that is a means to many ends, including stress management and the prevention and cure of many stress-related diseases. Though meditation is becoming quite a common practice for many people, there is still the misconception that it is complicated, mystical, and time-consuming. Actually, meditation is a very simple tool that can be learned in a few minutes and can be very beneficial even if practiced for only a few minutes a day. For an introduction to meditation, see "A Disciplined Mind through Meditation," on page 41.

YOGA SUTRA 2:53...
And the mind is prepared for steadiness.

Clarity

Along with striving for a disciplined mind, another aspect of a complete yoga practice is clarity, which in this case means having the ability to see things for what they really are. The founding practitioners of yoga emphasized the importance of having an honest, clear, and realistic view of the world and our place in it. Clarity frees us from the preconceptions, disappointments, and judgments that come from perceiving the world through either rose-colored glasses or unnecessary pessimism. It is achieved by being aligned with the truth. Clarity creates the foundation for honesty: Only when we acknowledge and accept things as they are can we communicate with ourselves and one another with accuracy and integrity.

In yoga, the term *authenticity* is used to describe the quality in a person that comes from acting from a place of clarity and connection with oneself. Yogis believe that one's external, physical life (i.e., status, goals, title, and actions) cannot be separated from one's inner life (i.e., thoughts, hopes, dreams, and sense of fulfillment). So being "authentic" in your life means fulfilling your individual potential, not trying to live up to others' expectations.

Our response to the world is often colored by stress and negativity or preconceived notions of reality. On top of that, we simply don't take the time to really look, listen, and taste. Mental chatter demands a lot of attention, and when our mind is overactive, we don't fully experience our senses. We achieve clarity when we can see the world without projecting ourselves, our expectations, and our moods onto our senses and perceptions, when we no longer pass every experience through the filter of our own perspective.

Simple meditative exercises can also be used to attain clarity. The following exercise works with literal vision, our eyesight. Sit in the basic meditation posture (see "A Disciplined Mind through Meditation," on page 41). Take several deep breaths. Soften your facial muscles, particularly those around your eyes and mouth. Relax your tongue and throat. Raise your fingertips to your temples, and with gentle pressure, massage in small circles until you feel tension melt away.

Next, think of softening your eyeball, as if releasing tension from inside the socket. Breathe deeply. Now, slowly open your eyes, and as you do so, imagine yourself absorbing what you see, as if it were coming to you. Don't force them to see anything. Let your vision come gradually into focus. Experience the color, texture, and shape of everything you see as if you've never seen such objects before. This is more an act of receiving than of research, so don't draw conclusions about what you see or try to define it. Stay open, receptive, and neutral. Continue to breathe deeply. Your intellect will probably strain to get involved in the act of seeing, but don't let it. Allow your senses to awaken on their own.

Continue your observation for several seconds until you feel your perceptions alter from hard and external to soft and internal. This simple exercise helps us integrate our inner and outer experiences. It stops us momentarily and asks us to reconsider our perceptions. It helps us understand the relationship between thinking and feeling. This is a nice way to start the day. Plan to do this in the morning, the first time you open your eyes.

Freedom

The third principle is freedom, the letting go of attachments. Yoga sees an attachment as something that is unhealthy, draining, and unproductive—a distraction that keeps you from your true purpose.

By heightening consciousness, yoga puts your focus on the present. Fear, anxiety, and feelings of inadequacy (these are all food triggers) are usually rooted in the baggage-heavy past or a hypothetical future. Vague, free-floating uneasiness is less likely to get hold of you if you're anchored securely within yourself, moment to moment.

Some examples of unhealthy attachments are indulgences in negative thinking, unhealthy relationships, and bad habits. They are weaknesses. Once you discipline the mind and look at the world with honesty, you will naturally let go of such attachments.

As part of your daily yoga practice, you'll also let go of the need to worry. Loosen your attachment to and your fear of things over which you have no control.

Anxiety solves nothing; it only causes stress and illness. Of course, not every fear you experience is unfounded. But yoga will help you decide which fears are rational and relevant to the present and guide you through the anxiety they cause you.

There are simple techniques that can be used to hone that power of discernment and facilitate the process of letting go. The following exercise is a good on-the-spot mechanism to use when you're seized by a negative feeling or a worry or when you find yourself in an incredibly stressful situation. It combines breathing with visualization.

First, remove yourself from the circumstances that have you feeling cornered. Whether it's traffic or a confrontation, you can take a minute and pull over or go into the next room. Give yourself about a minute of private time. Sit, stand, or lie down. Take a long, slow exhalation. Now begin breathing to a count. Inhale for one count, exhale for one count. Inhale for two counts, exhale for two counts. Inhale for three, exhale for three. Keep your breath smooth, steady, and soft. Don't try to force the air into or out of your lungs. As you exhale, imagine consciously releasing tension from your body. Imagine shifting your mind from high gear into neutral. This observation can help you slow down and gain perspective.

There's another great way to facilitate letting go. This exercise is more preventive and should help you keep things from getting hooked into you in the first place. It can be done first thing in the morning, right after the clarity exercise.

YOGA SUTRA 1:13...
The practice of yoga is the commitment to become established in the state of freedom.

Take 10 deep breaths and then state to yourself your focus for the day. If during either the 10 breaths or the vision exercise you find your mind getting attached to an anxiety, your statement for the day should be that you will accept the presence of that worry and realize your ability to deal with it. Remind yourself that you are doing your best and do your best to keep things in perspective.

Most people in the West initially approach yoga as a tool more for physical than for spiritual fitness—and with good reason. It strengthens and tones muscles, corrects posture and alignment, improves circulation to muscles and organs, streamlines bodily functions, teaches us how to breathe, calms the nervous system, reduces stress, and boosts energy. Nonetheless, the meditative focus on the breath generates emotional and spiritual benefits. An improved state of mind goes hand in hand with yoga's physical results: Free the body, and you free the mind.

Live with Integrity

This book will not tell you what to do for each meal or how to handle every day. You have to decide that. It is up to you to figure out the right things for your life and to do them. This strategy for well-being requires total integrity. Its most important prerequisite (and most significant result) is strength of character. It requires commitment, hard work, and honesty. No more self-lies; no more cheating—be it with diet pills and other quick fixes or with fatty, salty, low-nutrition shortcuts.

If you're going to take the position of being accountable for your life, you have to actively fill that role. Take on that responsibility for your life as if it's the greatest opportunity ever presented to you. This life is your big break. Go at it with all the focus, strength, determination, and precision that you would if it were a second chance at life—because it is. This strategy is not merely about management. It's about self-leadership.

Yoga brings forth the tools we need for living like leaders; it helps us find the skill necessary to take care of ourselves in such a busy world and to think outside the box we've been locked in. Our bodies are designed for survival. They are intended to stay alive and be as healthy as possible in any given environment. With yoga, you will discover and cultivate your instinctive desire for greater health and you will learn to stop sabotaging it.

If I tell you not to deprive yourself, you know as well as I do that this doesn't mean you should go eat an entire chocolate cake. If I say you should celebrate with food, you and I both know this isn't license to gorge. I may tell you that doing yoga before a party can act as damage control for the foods and drinks you may consume, but we both know this is not encouragement to binge after every session on the mat. You will get some terrific tools; it's up to you to use them consciously, not wastefully. As with any leader, do not use the power you are given for corrupt ends. True commitment takes integrity. Integrity is the product of being honest with yourself. The key to developing this practice is to discover and use your integrity.

When it comes down to it, the most important ingredient a person needs in order to implement change is discipline. Take the energy you usually direct at trying to control things you can't control and turn it toward your own behavior. You do have control over your thoughts, your decisions, your actions, and your reactions. Instead of worrying about the hypothetical future or trying to rein in the years, why not exercise a bit of self-discipline and self-leadership? It's time to stop being lazy and to start being honest. I know when I'm indulging in negative thinking or other lazy reflexes, and so do you. I'm the only one who can put an end to what will otherwise become a downward spiral on every level in my life. And I do. And so can you.

If we can overcome our social and psychological limitations and recover our spiritual nature, we can do our best in life. We can all be better people.

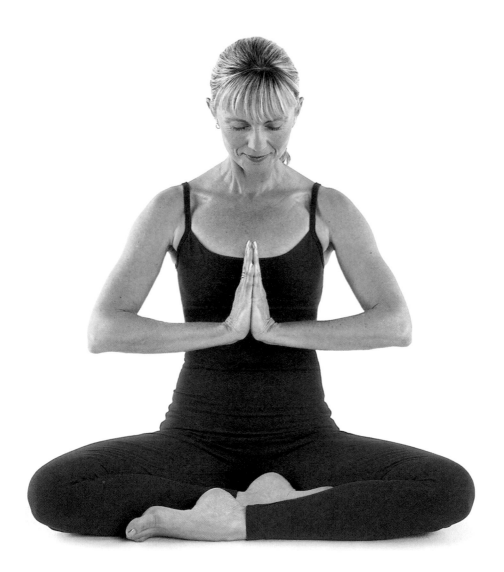

A Disciplined Mind through Meditation

To calm your mind, try the following: Sit on the floor in a cross-legged position. If this is uncomfortable for you due to tight hips or a stiff lower back, sit on a firmly folded blanket or a cushion or two—enough so that you are comfortable. You can also sit on a chair with your feet a comfortable distance apart and flat on the floor. Place your hands on your thighs.

Begin with a comfortably paced breath. Align yourself so that your spine is long from your tailbone upward though your head. Imagine your spine is suspended by a string that is connected toward the back of your head. This will naturally lengthen the back of your neck and slightly drop your chin. Your torso should feel spacious, not stiff.

Close your eyes. While maintaining your posture in a relaxed manner, turn your attention toward your breath. Notice its rhythm. To keep the focus inward, say to yourself with each breath, "I am inhaling breath" and "I am exhaling breath." You will probably notice after some time that your mind has wandered. Just bring it back and say again, "I am inhaling breath; I am exhaling breath."

When you can sit for several seconds with your mind focused on your breathing, return your attention to your posture. Most likely you will have fallen into a slump of some kind. Gently bring yourself back to the correct seated position and return your awareness to the breath. Continue to alternate your direct attention between the breath and your posture, without letting go of either.

The result of this is a focused, conscious state of mind. As your ability to concentrate and your strength improves, your whole body will feel bright, light, and warm. When body, mind, and breath are connected and immersed in the present moment, you will experience feeling whole and integrated. Like wiping a chalkboard clean of scribbles, lists, and problems to be solved, this practice helps to clear away the clutter and show the way to natural solutions and organic decisions.

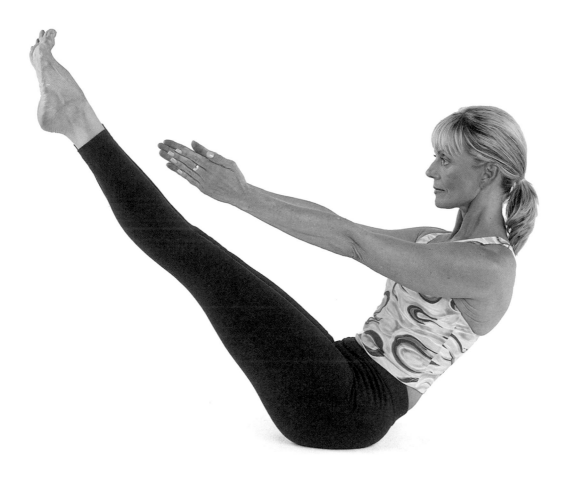

[3]

NUTRITION

All bodies are not the same, so I'm not going to tell you what to eat to lose weight. As you continue this practice, it will be up to you to establish a healthy program for your own body based on a new understanding of it. Your connection with yourself will serve to provide personalized guidelines for what you should eat and how much.

I hope to get you on the right track with essential background information about the delicate balance that exists between food and our bodies. This chapter will offer guidelines to help you reach a conscious and well-informed relationship with food. The most important initial step anyone can take in eating properly is to educate her/himself about food. While some of this will come from reading books and visiting doctors or health care specialists with an integrated health approach, it will also come from your own thoughtful investigation about different foods and how they effect you. In the process, you will explore the emotional motivations behind your food compulsions and discover some of the triggers for cravings and binges.

To further round out your knowledge and to form your own integrated perspective on health, look for resources about medical traditions such as Ayurvedic medicine from India and Chinese medicine. These disciplines use a holistic approach to the body and mind that complements the Western medical tradition.

Convenience-Food Nation

Convenience practically founded this country. Our ancestors were so busy on their way to the frontier, so busy founding a new civilization, that they didn't have time for nice meals. Food as a civilized, nurturing concept flew out the window. It may have been reestablished with the family dinner at some point, but it flew out the window again with our current pursuit of new financial frontiers.

Convenience is the motor driving development in American culture, and it extends to our attitudes about everything we do: shopping, the environment, child rearing, relationships, conversation, cooking, and eating.

We eat on the run. We eat in the car. We buy frozen food in a box, push a button, and *presto!* We eat lunch at our desks while we multitask—and that's if we decide to have a meal at all. Why not just snack all day?

When they can't make it sound good, frozen-, fast-, and snack-food companies make food sound fun, which leads me to our next downfall. People have nearly forgotten what food is for. Go to the nearest airport or train station, where there are people waiting. Just around the corner, there will undoubtedly be long lines and a herd of people with plastic trays eating chili dogs, and they're doing it because they have nothing else to do. We eat when we are bored, and we usually do it without thinking. We eat out of habit just because the food is there. Food is no longer about nourishment; it's about distraction.

Pizza is not a pastime. Eating this way doesn't show any respect for our bodies or health, or for life in general. Food used to be something people either rejoiced for or rejoiced with. They celebrated this thing that sustained the miracle of life. We need to cultivate this attitude. If we move through life with awareness, if we take time to think consciously, it may occur to us to pack our own healthy snacks and meals for the airport or for lunch at our desks.

It might occur to us to think about the way food really tastes and how it makes us feel. I guarantee this simple change would play a significant role in shaping a new future for you and your health.

The Lure of the Quick Fix

Does the world really need more temporary solutions? Our culture consistently tries to make up for its excess with shortcut gimmicks that claim to save time: fast food, the snack frenzy, weight loss pills, caffeine instead of sleep, even e-mail and the Internet. Does e-mail really save time? Doesn't it just allow you to do more, faster?

In terms of dieting, years of one quick fix after another have probably done nothing to give you the body you were pining for. If you had only decided long ago to make a healthy lifestyle change, you would have lasting results by now, and years of feeling good about yourself under your belt. It's not too late to make that change.

People who are "thin" thanks to cabbage-soup regimens, stomach stapling, or diet pills are not necessarily healthy. It's a constant struggle, going from one trick to the next, and it's harmful to your system. Yo-yo dieters are left with slow metabolism, poor nutrition, fatigue, and low self-esteem. Long-term dieting has a negative impact on a person's faith in his or her ability to succeed and can lead to obsessive diets that amount to slow starvation. A weight fixation easily slips across the line to become an eating disorder.

Where do we get this idea that we all have to be a size 2? It's everywhere. It may come from magazines and movies, but it may also be an inverse reaction to the growing number of obese people. We've got to start from scratch in our attitudes about food. When you begin to think of food with respect, you consider it as fuel and look at it in terms of ecological balance and healthful living. As you do so, your diet will change—out of respect both for what you put in your mouth and how your body will react to it. The foods you will turn to instinctively will actually work to recalibrate your system and establish balance to your body and your weight. We need to backtrack with our diets, our way of life, and return to what's essential.

The Truth about "Diet" Foods

Today's medical research supports the fact that a diet rich in fruits and vegetables, low in fat, and adequate in protein can prevent heart disease, cancer, digestive disorders, and diabetes—all of which are rampant in our country. No matter what the disease, nutritionists will tell you, inadequate or inappropriate food and insufficiency of both micro- and macronutrients play a significant role in illness. But as with so many things, knowledge seems to have done little to change behavior.

In our country, we have an incredibly conflicted relationship with food. It's no surprise that we are caught in epidemics of both obesity and diabetes. These diseases are products of our lifestyle and are exacerbated by overeating, skipping meals, excessive dieting, refined foods, and lack of exercise. Many of us don't pay attention to how we eat, what we eat, or how much we eat.

Those among us who do try to watch our waistlines have gotten the wrong message and think that fat-free ''foods'' are the answer, replacing natural whole foods with no-fat frozen dinners, cookies, yogurts, ice creams, potato chips, and other products containing fat substitutes. It may surprise you to learn that people who eat this stuff are gaining more weight than anyone else! These foods are often based on chemicals, loaded with sugar or sodium, and low in nutritional value. When they're not high in sugar, they are high in sugar substitutes that are difficult to digest and have been shown to cause cancer in laboratory animals.

One of the biggest dangers of fat-free products—and one that diet-food manufacturers capitalize on—is that our minds trick us into believing that it's okay to eat larger quantities. If the chips are fat-free, we rationalize, why shouldn't we eat a whole bag? Unfortunately, there is no such thing as a free lunch—even if it is *fat*-free. Our bodies can be challenged by processed foods, especially in large quantities, and eating them causes digestive disturbances. Proper and efficient digestion is a cornerstone to maintaining a healthy weight.

These foods do have calories, no matter how hard they try not to, but they're "empty" calories, lacking nutritional value. Eating such foods is a complete waste of calories—it's like buying something you don't need just because it's on sale. You still spend more money than you would have if it hadn't been on sale and you hadn't bought it. It would be healthier to have a small, satisfying serving of real ice cream when you really want it than a pint of fat-free frozen yogurt every day. There are wonderful naturally rich foods with appropriate fat content in the world, such as organic raw nuts, avocados, eggs, goat cheese, and real yogurt. Find them and your body will learn to like them.

A typical "low-fat" diet for someone on the run includes "meals" that feature lots of bread topped with fat-free cream cheese, low-fat peanut butter, or another butter substitute; tuna salad with mayonnaise (fat-free or regular); cottage cheese, yogurt, or frozen yogurt with toppings like canned fruits, granola, nuts, or M&Ms; snacks such as pretzels, popcorn, energy bars, and diet cookies; diet soda, coffee with cream or milk, milk powder, sugar, or sugar substitutes. On top of this, these busy, malnourished folks eat in their car or at their desk, on the phone, or while walking down the sidewalk. I know weight-conscious people eat this way, and I know they think it's healthy. They think it's the best they can do for their bodies, that it's the best they can do to lose weight or keep their weight down.

These dieters are either fooling themselves or they are misled. We've been taught that this is a healthy diet. It's not. This diet is not balanced—it is high in dairy; laden with sugar and carbohydrates, refined additives, and chemically derived substitutes; and low in fiber, nutrition, flavor, and variety.

Another dieter's pitfall: immense servings of "low-fat" meals loaded with toppings that are overdosed with flavoring. The "healthy" chef's salad usually presents a logger's portion of processed ham, turkey, and cheese, drenched in salad dressing—oh, yeah, and a few greens. The chicken Caesar salad, though delicious, is also hardly a dieter's choice, with its Parmesan cheese (often not the real thing), egg, stale and greasy croutons, extremely salty (and often high-fat) dressing, and loads of chicken—and a few greens. Another "healthy" option is the famous baked potato with butter, sour cream, "bacon" bits, Cheddar cheese, and more. By the time you make your way through the toppings on any of these healthy meals, you'll consume more calories (and chemicals) than if you had eaten grilled chicken or salmon with vegetables. And you're shocking your taste buds into ineffectiveness. Tongues of condiment lovers have become so accustomed to sodium and sugar, everything else seems bland by comparison. The essence of the real food is lost under those saucy concoctions.

Learn to enjoy the taste of simple food, to distinguish the subtleties of your palate. Brown rice has a meaty aroma. Potatoes are rich. Carrots, peppers, and most vegetables are sweet—especially if they are organic and fresh. Try them steamed.

As your connection with your body is established and your senses awaken, your ability to taste will be enhanced. It is essential to think of food as an integral part of a holistic lifestyle, to respect it as you respect nature and love it as you love your life. Gratitude and respect come from making a conscious effort toward something. But all too often, Americans don't think we have to work for our food. We just put something in the microwave for two minutes, then shove it in our mouths for two minutes, and call that a meal. The least you can do before you eat a meal is to think about it.

What Price Convenience?

Our bodies are faced with many chemical triggers, including stress and pollution, that combine to create imbalances within. Consumption of certain things also causes a series of hormonal and chemical chain reactions in the body. Refined foods, which include sugar and white flour, have a similar affect. Our bodies may react unpredictably during the digestive process when they encounter something that does not originate in nature. We are not biologically designed to recognize a cheese crisp as nourishment because it's not. Our bodies' response to it is, "What is this thing?! Attention all systems: foreign matter!" When we eat one, our immune system kicks in because its job is to deal with unidentifiable things, or invaders, in the body. This is a waste of the body's resources, and over time it wears us down.

Refined foods also lead to overproduction of insulin (the hormone that regulates glucose and metabolizes fat), which is a major culprit in heart disease, diabetes, and irregular levels of glucose. Difficulty losing weight is often tied to insulin resistance, as having too much insulin in the bloodstream inhibits the breakdown of fat by the body. Everything we eat affects insulin production. On the bright side, this means it is the only hormone in the body over which we have some degree of control.

Eat as few refined and processed products as possible. Whole, natural foods produce a realistic insulin response. Their digestion releases just the right amount of insulin to do its job on a cellular level. After we eat refined foods or imbalanced foods (such as simple sugars, hydrogenated oils, or synthetic fats), too much insulin is produced, saturating our cells. The excess insulin stays in the bloodstream because it has no place else to go. If insulin is inhibited from doing its job, fat collects in the bloodstream and in the body. (The same thing happens when we skip meals. Think twice the next time you forgo breakfast to cut calories; it will actually make you a fat sponge.) This leads not only to diabetes and obesity but also to heart disease.

As we get fat and sick, we get sad, and it's not just because of the way we look and feel. One of insulin's jobs is to regulate glucose, or blood sugar. Glucose is brain food, and its levels in our bodies affect our mental capacity and our emotions. Low blood sugar leaves us feeling disoriented; high blood sugar leaves us overstimulated and unfocused. Balanced blood sugar helps us feel centered. If insulin can't bring glucose to the cells, we suffer from hypoglycemia, symptoms of which include memory problems, depression, and fatigue. This is a perfect example of the lowest state of mind in yogic thought, the dull or lethargic mind, being a result of a physical imbalance.

Refined, processed foods have been stripped of nutritional value. That includes most canned, preserved, pickled, bottled, bleached, polished, dyed, and refined foods. It includes baked goods made with white flour and preservatives or fat substitutes. It includes high-sugar baked goods, like most muffins. It even includes most diet and energy bars. If you have to choose between one of these and a bag of chips, use your instincts. Read the label and choose the option with the most recognizable natural ingredients and the fewest unpronounceable words. (A good rule of thumb: If a food's list of ingredients gets beyond four ingredients or five syllables, you might not want to put that food in your mouth.)

It is possible to find healthy, organic canned foods, and they are worth looking for. You can have some of the convenience of not having to shop quite as often without having to sacrifice nutrition completely. If possible, every meal should be based on whole, natural foods. Canned or frozen foods should be limited to one side dish in a meal.

Don't get sucked in by marketing. Health bars, fruit juice smoothies, or so-called "protein shakes" blast our bodies with sugar and carbohydrates and don't provide much in the way of fiber. *Eat real food.* If you need the nutrients in orange juice, eat an orange. If you need protein, eat a handful of raw almonds.

One more thing: Become a conscious snacker. Most snacks are junk food. If you consistently get hungry between meals, eat smaller meals at breakfast, lunch, and dinner and supplement with midday minimeals (healthy snacks) of fresh fruits and vegetables, yogurt, grains, or a handful of nuts. Some people do better with the standard three square meals; others prefer the five-small-meals format. Figure out which works for you.

A New Relationship with Food

Yoga has taught for ages that food plays an important role in health and well-being and that it plays a significant role in overcoming and even preventing mental and physical illness—something our culture is only beginning to come to terms with.

Yogis believe that food can affect us in three ways: It can provide nourishment, energy, and strength; it can be the source of mental distress; or it can impede bodily functions and lead to physical illness. If food can have an unhealthy effect on our bodies, it will also have an unhealthy impact on our minds.

We can't always control what we are served. At a party or a restaurant, you don't want to drive the hostess, waiter, or other guests crazy with special dietary requests, but you can choose to eat more of the healthful choices available and a smaller portion of those things that you know will cause you problems later.

Practicing yoga will help to build a steady emotional and intellectual relationship with food. Because it makes us stop, look, and listen to our bodies instead of just reacting and counterreacting mentally and physically, yoga can break the unhealthy relationships that exist among food, emotions, and body chemistry and help us regain control over our systems. Let your body lead you down the path to health with a diet that's really right for you.

Yoga has always been connected with a diet that would reflect its core beliefs. Because yoga teaches a respect for life that extends to all living things, and because yoga originated in Hindu India, where people don't eat meat, the classic yogic diet is traditionally vegetarian with an emphasis on fresh fruits and vegetables, milk, butter, beans, honey, cereals, and water; the body's needs for protein and fat are met by a significant daily portion of dairy products and legumes. The traditional, completely vegetarian, high-dairy diet may not be relevant for everyone today because of increasing chemical sensitivities to dairy products and because our busy lives may make meat a necessary part of a healthy diet. But it is a good model to follow and make adaptations to. The bulk of one's diet is comprised of grains, fruits and vegetables, and legumes. Meat should play a secondary role, as a side dish to a main meal. Whether someone chooses to eat dairy and meat would depend on how his or her body responds; if you do eat dairy or meat, do everything you can to choose organic dairy products and hormone-free meats.

Where Do I Begin?

The best approach would be to use your body's innate tools and combine that awareness with a diet based on the classic yogic diet. Again, a completely vegetarian diet may not be the best choice for everyone, especially with the physical and emotional demands we face in our daily lives. When I began studying yoga as a life path, I wanted to pursue the yogic lifestyle 100 percent and adopted the traditional diet. I was a vegetarian for years, and for years, I felt hungry. Eventually, I incorporated small amounts of fish and chicken into my diet and the constant hunger was gone. Remember: If you want to adopt a vegetarian lifestyle, try it, but make the change slowly, educate yourself in advance, and listen to your body.

Meat, in small portions, is not inherently unhealthy, and most people need the nutrients that can be found only in meat. Vegetarians usually choose not to eat meat for two reasons: First, the meat industry's inhumane treatment of animals raised for consumption runs counter to practicing respect for all life; and second, most meat is treated heavily with hormones and antibiotics. When we eat that meat, we ingest those hormones and antibiotics. Though meat in gross quantities has been shown to increase the incidence of heart disease, it is generally agreed that small portions of meat are a great nutritional complement to meals based largely on vegetables, grains, and beans. Your stomach is about the size of the palm of your hand; portions should not greatly outsize your fist.

One way to exercise the yogic approach and still eat meat is to seek organic, hormone-free, farm-raised meats and fresh fish. When shopping for organic, hormone- and antibiotic-free meats, read labels carefully and do your research. There are varying degrees of "hormone-free" and "low antibiotic." For example, a lot of meat sold as "hormone-free" comes from animals that were treated with hormones for the first three months of their lives.

A word about dairy products: Unfortunately, they are also often quite heavily treated with hormones and antibiotics and chemically altered by the process of pasteurization. Some doubt that the calcium in pasteurized, homogenized, hormone-infused milk can be recognized and absorbed by our bodies, but they have yet to be proven right or wrong. Though the question of calcium absorption is unsettled, we do know that recombinant bovine growth hormone (rbGH), which is in a lot of nonorganic dairy products, is bad news for humans. It has been linked to several disorders, including premature menstruation, behavioral problems like attention deficit disorder, and possibly even hormone-induced cancers.

Sensitivity to cow's milk is becoming common, especially in people with asthma or other allergies. Some find that goat's milk, goat cheese, and goat yogurt are easier to digest and produce fewer allergy symptoms. Goat's milk is more like human milk than cow's milk is. It's allergen-free, and with 10 grams of carbohydrates and 9 grams of protein per serving, it's a nicely balanced food. If you do have reactions to dairy, give the goat dairy products a try. As always, keep an eye out for an organic brand. Soy is also a great dairy replacement. Look for calcium-rich organic soy milk and yogurt. Other great sources of calcium are almonds, sesame seeds, spinach, and kale.

Nuts and grains are a great food source—particularly if they are raw and unsalted. In ancient times when nomadic tribes crossed deserts by foot, they carried little more than nuts and grains to eat. Explorers at the turn of the last century did the same. They would survive for months in arduous conditions on trail mix and pemmican (dried meat). Just remember, chances are you're burning up less energy than a man crossing the Sahara or the Arctic by foot; one little handful at a time is enough for a snack.

If white bagels are such a big deal in your diet that you can't imagine breakfast without them, you're in a food rut. Try a thin, dense slice of wheat-free, 100 percent natural pumpernickel or linseed bread with a little butter and some honey for a change. Or real oatmeal cooked slowly with a bit of nutmeg, cloves, and cardamom. Or goat yogurt with fresh fruit sliced into it. Or baked apples with cinnamon. Or a hard-boiled egg, a slice of turkey, and a plum. You have some great options.

Variety is a very healthy dietary cornerstone. Overuse of any one food is not good for your body. If you eat too much wheat, your body will get saturated with it and your system will go into over-drive and develop an intolerance for it. The same thing happens with casein and lactose, found in dairy products. Take a two-to-three-day holiday from any food you find yourself eating consistently, and rotate which foods you're taking a break from.

YOGA SUTRA 1:33...
The mind becomes clear and serene
when the qualities of the heart
are cultivated.

Nutrition Tips

* Learn to listen to your body. Know when you are full and do not overeat.

* Be mindful of your breathing while you are eating.

* Chew your food. Chewing stimulates the digestive juices in the mouth necessary for proper digestion, which will help your food be absorbed by your body for fuel.

* Notice which foods make you feel satisfied and give you energy and which foods make you feel tired, bloated, sluggish, or stuffy.

* Plan your meals. Think about fueling your body and nourishing yourself.

* Take your time eating. Rushing induces the cortisol reaction and insulin resistance, as well as increasing food sensitivities and cravings.

* Eat fresh vegetables when you can. Also, keep a variety of fresh frozen vegetables in the freezer. These have better nutritional value than canned vegetables and make for a quick, tasty, and healthy complement to a meal.

* Eat a variety of foods and try new ones. Encourage your metabolism by eating a varied diet including green vegetables, whole grains, fresh fruits, olive oil, nuts, fish, and small portions of poultry and meat.

* Choose foods in harmony with the seasons. This will ensure their freshness.

* Learn to use herbs and exotic spices to season your foods. Your taste buds will be delighted and they have many healthful effects.

* Make friends with healthy fat. It satiates you and improves your complexion. Go for healthy fats, such as those found in olive oil, salmon, avocado, fresh nuts, and real yogurt, in small portions.

* Always have your salad dressing on the side and use it sparingly. Taste the vegetables, not the topping.

* If you have the opportunity to choose between real butter and margarine for spreading or cooking, always go for butter and use it sparingly.

* Avoid processed foods.

* Avoid nondairy creamer and artificial sweeteners.

* Avoid soft drinks, even diet soft drinks. Most of them contain aspartame, which has been shown to inhibit the body's ability to lose weight. Also, the carbonation in soda has been linked to osteoporosis.

* Avoid foods cooked in sauces, but if you must, have the sauce on the side and use it sparingly.

* If you eat in restaurants, choose the simple dishes that follow the vegetable/whole grain/fish, poultry, or meat example.

* Order or cook your poultry, meat, or fish grilled, broiled, or baked.

* Drink plenty of fresh water. If it becomes boring, flavor it with a squeeze of lemon or lime.

* As a healthy substitute for sugar, use stevia, an herb that can be found in most health-food stores in powdered bulk form or as a liquid in a bottle. Stevia is 30 times sweeter than sugar, so you just need a pinch, and it has no aftertaste. It has been shown to help regulate blood sugar.

* Make changes in your diet consciously and don't go cold turkey. Cutting out everything all at once will only cause you to feel deprived, which often leads to bingeing.

Focus on Whole Foods

Large-scale marketing campaigns have led us to believe on one hand that food is entertainment and on the other hand that food is the enemy. It's time to return to basics with an emphasis on whole, natural foods as vital and pleasurable. It's also time to remember that food is fuel for the body.

Our bodies have a wisdom that predates this society and its products. Our genetic, biological program was mapped out centuries ago, before food came in boxes and cans. Perhaps the best trick to maintaining a balanced relationship with food is one of the most obvious: Eat natural foods. The closer the food on our plates comes to resembling the way it's found in nature, the easier it will be recognized and digested by our bodies. These high-tech foods are foreign to our digestive systems. That's why their consumption induces chemical reactions in the body, like insulin resistance, low glucose levels, and cortisol inflammation. These in turn lead to another set of problems, from poor digestion, low metabolism, cravings, and allergies to diabetes, depression, obesity, and heart disease.

The body is able to recover. Our goal is to help you rethink your diet so your body once again knows what to do with the food you're feeding it. All it takes is a return to nature and balance. You've seen those lucky people who seem to eat almost anything they want, never overeat or diet, and don't seem to have a conflicted or obsessive relationship with food. That can be you.

Cultivate a calm, nurturing connection with food. Healthy eating is not about deprivation. It's about abundance. Real meals of natural foods leave you feeling sated, balanced, and taken care of. Realistic portions of whole foods improve digestion, encourage insulin sensitivity, increase metabolism, help burn fat, and decrease cravings. With this approach, binges would fall by the wayside. You would look and feel a hundred times better. More importantly, you would get more joy out of life.

Stop playing games and start nourishing yourself. A natural-food diet with variety and moderation can include foods we've been told are off-limits, even butter and chocolate. But it also makes these foods less important because they will always be an option. Remember, yoga is about celebrating life; life is about feeling open and lively. It's not about restrictions. Eat a variety of foods, but eat in moderation. Walk the middle path. It may seem too simple, but it works. Real food has always worked to sustain life and health, and it still will.

Pay Attention to Your Body

Where do you start? Pay attention to how you feel when you eat. Remember, this is what food is for: to maintain life. It should stimulate and energize you. People think the "food coma" is a normal part of the digestive process, but a meal shouldn't tire you out. Do you feel alive after a meal, or do you feel bloated and heavy? Does your stomach hurt? Does your mouth get dry or your breath stink? Do you consistently cough or get stuffy when you eat cheese, or get an itchy mouth after a peanut butter sandwich? Do you get rashes and night sweats after certain meals? Do some foods only make you want to eat more and more of that food? Do some things make you sleepy? Reactions such as these can be signs of a food intolerance or food allergy. Even someone with no history of an allergy to wheat or dairy products can develop one, especially in times of stress or when exposed to pollutants or other allergens.

Stress is reportedly one of the biggest factors underlying food sensitivities or allergies. Our crazy lives affect our body chemistry. As part of an innate defense system, our bodies produce chemicals under duress. Unfortunately, many of them cause inflammation and increase the body's sensitivity. Rushing around, overdoing it, and worrying increase the level of cortisol and its sidekick, an inflammatory chemical called interleukin-6, in the body. These natural chemicals can increase your sensitivity and cause you to react badly to everything from pollen and pollution to gluten, dairy, and wheat. Often, one sensitivity leads to another. If you have a lot of food sensitivities, look closely at how you manage the stress in your life.

These chemicals do more than cause swelling or irritation. Cortisol feels like adrenaline or a caffeine high. It makes you feel as if you're moving fast in a straight line but have no idea where to. (This is a symptom of the distracted and scattered states of mind, as discussed in Chapter 1, and is an example of how a physical state can lead to a mental imbalance.) By blocking glucose, cortisol affects memory (it is a potential player behind our "mental blocks"), and by inhibiting serotonin, it affects our moods. Serotonin is a naturally produced feel-good chemical, the effects of which can be induced by exercise as well as proper nutrition. A lot of overweight people are depressed and are put on antianxiety drugs and antidepressants. These may help, but so might tracking food intolerance and eliminating the things in their diets that they can't effectively digest.

If you think you don't have food allergies, see what happens after you've started to clean out the clutter in your body and replace it with proper food and exercise. By eating healthfully, you will enhance your body's ability to raise flags at certain foods. Pay attention to those alerts: Your body can convey extremely valuable information if you listen.

Our bodies' chain reaction is significant in terms of overeating and weight gain because the immune response in an allergic reaction can be a catalyst to food cravings, and the chemical response itself inhibits our ability to process fat. Ask yourself what you crave. It's usually exactly the thing you shouldn't be eating, the food you have an allergy to. Try steering clear of it for a while, and the craving for it will probably go away. One typical example of this is the person "addicted" to bread (and probably reacting to refined flour) or candy (reacting to refined sugar). As soon as they wean themselves off bread or candy, they don't crave it any more.

Your overeating triggers may be chemical and/or emotional, and by avoiding them, you can improve the state of your body, mind, and spirit.

Tools for Finding Balance

Again, what should be obvious isn't always. Simplicity may be the hardest thing for us to achieve in our lives. We don't live in a world that supports a purely whole-foods lifestyle. We honestly don't always have time to make sure there's a balanced meal in the fridge, fresh and ready to eat. Most of us don't have the luxury of shopping every day and need the convenience of canned tomatoes, canned beans, and so on.

Remember to keep your expectations realistic. You're not expected to become a subsistence farmer of organic fruits and vegetables, nor is that necessary to live a healthy life. Just thinking about food as something that should come from nature will engender a healthy change in your choices. Most large grocery stores do have an organic health-food aisle. If the foods there seem more expensive, keep in mind that you won't be spending as much on bagged or canned snacks like potato chips, popcorn, and soda. Buy brown rice in bulk and eat in moderation, and you may find that you're spending less. Snack foods are expensive.

As I said earlier, ask yourself consciously whether you really want or need to eat what you're about to put in your mouth. Consider how it will make you feel. This will play a large part in healthy decision-making.

Getting real joy out of food is also essential to striking a balance. Health is not about deprivation. Food in all its variety is a wonderful expression of abundance. This does not have to run counter to moderation.

Life is about enjoyment. It's about a richness of experience. To practice a yogic approach to life is to be conscious of these things and to use them to connect to the natural world around you. Just as you've been given a body and should move it, you've also been given taste buds. Use them to try new things. We get into food ruts where we eat the same four things in different combinations for months or even years on end. We do so out of convenience or boredom or lack of time and creativity. Buy a cookbook and explore newness. Invite people over and share what you discover. I have a friend who constantly entertains and who always says, "Food is love." It is, in the sense that when we have a healthy relationship with food, it is nurturing, empowering, exciting and fulfilling, and it's something we can extend to others.

What you can do, no matter where you live or how much time you have, is to make whole foods the cornerstone of your diet. Incorporate whole foods into every meal. If you have to use canned beans, season them with fresh organic peppers, tomatoes, and farm-raised chicken. Get over the hurdle that assumes a home-cooked meal has to take hours to prepare. A dish of salmon steamed on a bed of vegetables takes about 10 minutes to prepare, surely less time than it would take to go to the closest restaurant, order, and wait.

You know what works for your body. If you don't know it intellectually, your body knows it biologically. Listen to your body. Trust your instincts—they are intended for survival and health. Let your body teach your mind. If you come from generations of overweight people, think outside that box. Redefine yourself. Be honest about why you may be heavy, what habits have gotten your family to where it is. Most fat families eat like fat families, with high-fat foods, snacks, sauces, and big portions. Be the one to break the chain.

Also, when making your food choices, think of your connection to the world. You are making a decision that shows a respect for all life and supports a way of living that encourages life. Organic foods are better for you, but they are also better for the rest of the world.

Balance self-accountability with compassion. You're trying. You're doing your best. You do know the solution, but it doesn't always come easily. If you find that a week's gone by and you've been going the convenience-food route or giving in to cravings instead of learning from them, just remember, this is only one week in your life. Move on!

A Word on Fasting

Fasting has long played a role in the traditional yogic diet. For people with busy lives, a true fast is probably not a good idea, even if it is just for one day. But healthy individuals can give their digestive systems a rest from carbohydrates, fat, and protein by rotating foods, as discussed earlier, or by doing a fruit-and-vegetable fast for a day—but not more than once a month. A 24-hour partial fast once a month is believed to rejuvenate the body by facilitating removal of waste from the bowels, kidneys, skin, and lungs and to purify the mind. Fasting of any kind is never recommended for individuals with anorexia, bulimia, diabetes, or kidney disorders or for people who've recently undergone detoxification programs for drugs and alcohol. Before embarking on a fast, speak with a qualified health care professional.

If you decide to do a gentle vegetable fast for a day, be sure to drink plenty of water with lemon and honey in it. This is a great liver and lymphatic cleanser and best taken first thing in the morning on an empty stomach. Just add the juice from half a lemon and $\frac{1}{2}$ teaspoon of honey to a cup of lukewarm water. This and an apple would be a good start to the day. Eat plenty of green, leafy vegetables with a low glycemic index (low sugar content) and high fiber. Rest, stretch lightly from time to time, focus on the breath, and take easy walks.

When finished, break the fast lightly. Slowly introduce gently cooked whole grains to your system, served with steamed or baked fruits and vegetables. At breakfast, for example, have a cooked pear in a bowl of soy milk with half a slice of flourless linseed bread. Lunch and dinner could include a sweet potato, a bit of brown rice, and steamed collard greens; or a hearty soup with vegetables and beans. Eat slowly and listen to your body. Chances are, you'll feel alert and rested, as if you've had a little vacation.

Part Two: The Yoga Practice

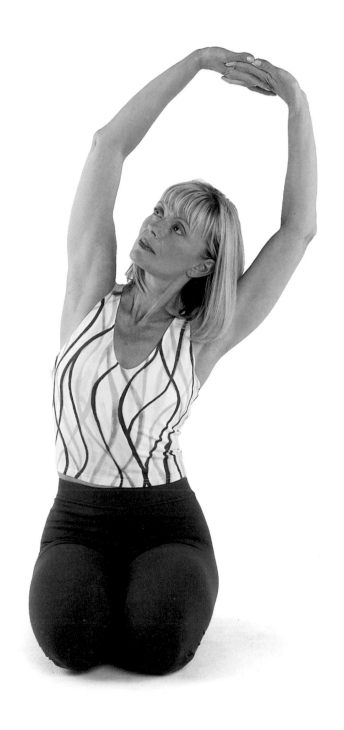

[4]

GETTING STARTED

Now that we know why yoga works and how to maintain its gifts in the face of a complex world, how to prepare our attitude, and how to properly nourish ourselves, let's move forward. In the second half of this book, we will get to the practical basics: the postures and breath, as well as reaffirming exercises to make your journey a more stable and enlightened one.

Yoga is a powerful practice that will change your life. It begins deep inside at the cellular level and works its way out. It shows up in your increased energy level, the glow of your skin, the light in your eyes, the calm in your voice, the shape of your body, and the ease and grace with which you move through your life.

Practicing yoga regularly helps to unravel the complexities of the mind. The *asanas* penetrate into each layer of the body and ultimately into the consciousness. This leads us to the realization that inspiration, peace, and happiness cannot come from the outside but must be cultivated and realized from within.

Things to Know

The yoga we will practice in this book is known as *hatha* yoga, an umbrella term covering many different practices. *Hatha*, which means "sun and moon," focuses on achieving a balance between the *yin* and *yang* energies of our bodies. This balance is the key to yoga and perhaps its most important result. The different kinds of *hatha* yoga— some examples include *Ashtanga, Iyengar, kundalini,* and *viniyoga*—and all have the same aim, but they get there by different means.

Our practice is based on the Iyengar approach, developed by B. K. S. Iyengar. Iyengar hatha yoga emphasizes precise postural alignment. Iyengar believes that through correct anatomical alignment in each posture, one can restore proper energy flow and bring the body and mind into balance. His method is well known for its incorporation of props such as foam bricks, straps, blankets, and wedges, which allow people of all levels of fitness to modify the postures and maintain correct alignment during the practice. Iyengar believes that the *pranayamas* (controlled breathing exercises) should be done separately from the *asanas* (postures), and should be introduced to the practice only after the student has mastered the basics.

Each person has physical strengths and weaknesses that work to compensate for each other. For instance, you may have very strong hamstring muscles and very weak (or overly flexible) quadriceps muscles. This imbalance may result in difficulties with the tendons in the knee. If tight hamstrings outpower the knee tendons, you need to lengthen, or stretch, the hamstrings and build up the quadriceps muscles. A single pose, when performed with the correct alignment, can help you achieve both things and, over time, establish a healthy give-and-take between the muscles' functions. The sequencing of postures in this yoga practice enhances and combines balance, flexibility, and strength.

Creating a Space

Your yoga practice is especially for you and will be one of the most enjoyable parts of your day. Give some thought to creating an inviting space in which to practice. The space you choose for your practice should make you feel peaceful and happy. Choose an area or a room that is quiet, simple, and clean. The size is not important, as long as you can stand upright and lay on the floor with your arms outstretched over your head and to your sides without bumping into anything. The floor should be uncarpeted, or carpeted very thinly, to give you a firm foundation. The temperature should be comfortable and the space should be well ventilated, not drafty. It's also nice to create ambience before you begin. Some people like to play soothing music during practice; others mist the air with their favorite aromatherapy spray, light a candle, or burn incense. Wherever you practice, turn your phone off!

Equipment

To practice yoga, you will need a lightweight yoga mat with a nonslip surface. (New sticky mats are sometimes slippery! Your new yoga mat can be lightly cleaned with a nonabrasive, nontoxic cleaner. Use a damp sponge or cloth with a small amount of cleaner to remove any coating that may have been applied during manufacturing.) This will help keep your hands and feet in place, giving you a reliable anchor and a bit of firm cushion.

Most people benefit from the use of additional props: two foam yoga bricks, a yoga strap, and a blanket. These items are used throughout the practice and ensure that you maintain proper alignment by assisting you to correctly modify the postures according to your body. (Props can be found in most large department stores and sportswear stores, or online.) A chair can be used at the end of the practice to elevate your legs for deeper relaxation.

You should wear clothing that is comfortable. A T-shirt and loose-fitting pants or shorts with an elastic waist are great, as is cotton/spandex yoga wear, as long as it's not too tight! (Stay away from clothing that is 100 percent synthetic.) Yoga is always practiced with bare feet to enhance the connection of the body to the earth.

Pranayama

Most of us take breathing for granted and have never given much thought to doing it better. This is a drastic oversight. We work on our health and protect our well-being in many ways, but most people are shallow breathers. They are cheating themselves of oxygen the same way a chronic dieter cheats him- or herself of nutrients.

Without breath, life would not be. It nourishes the blood, the muscles, and the organs. The breath is a powerful and direct link to the nervous system. In simplified terms, our inhalation inspires and uplifts us, while our exhalation soothes and relaxes.

Try this exercise. Take a long, slow, deep inhalation. Fill your lungs from the bottom to the top. Feel your chest rise. Notice how your mind becomes absorbed in the process. Exhale slowly, smoothly, consistently, and as deeply as possible until your lungs are completely empty of air, without forcing it out. Feel your body and your mind relax as you release the pressure from your lungs. You will notice that after a few conscious breaths, your state of mind will change. You may feel more awake and present. You will release tension you didn't even know you were storing in your body!

Classic yogic breathing is called *pranayama*. In Sanskrit, *prana* means "breath of life." *Pranayama* is the rhythmic, conscious control of the breath through a variety of complex breathing patterns. The first step toward understanding *pranayama* is learning to keep a smooth, steady, rhythmic inhalation and exhalation while on the yoga mat. This means that you should always be aware of your breath while practicing yoga and that you should never force your body to do anything that would interrupt your smooth, steady pace. One way to heighten awareness of your breath throughout your day is to periodically count each inhalation and exhalation and try to keep them equal in duration.

For the poses in this book, we will use a simple breathing pattern. Inhale and exhale through your nose for 5 to 10 breaths for each pose. Do a count of 5 to start with and increase as you become better able to hold your attention on your breath and alignment. As your body begins to understand each pose, your breath will naturally increase in length; the time it will take for you to take 5 breaths will increase considerably in six months.

Generally speaking, you inhale to prepare for a posture and exhale as you move into it. Once there, use your breath to keep your mind focused on how you are feeling inside. Your inhalation has a lengthening and widening effect on your body, and for this reason, it is an inherent part of any stretching exercise. It enhances your ability to feel tightness in your muscles and naturally deepens your pose without force. It also keeps your mind alert. Use your inhalation to guide you gently into a deeper connection with yourself.

Your exhalation has a relaxing effect upon your mind and your body. While in your pose, exhale through your nose in a long, smooth, steady stream while maintaining the correct postural alignment. Working in this way allows the posture to strengthen your body, relax your nervous system, and focus your mind. This play of body, mind, and breath creates an internal awareness and cultivates the mind-body connection that is the foundation of the practice.

Off the mat, you will become more conscious of your breath. You might realize that your breathing is shallow or that you are unconsciously holding your breath for several seconds at a time. If so, just return to the rhythmic inhalation and exhalation of your practice. You will notice the beneficial yogic effects of breathing correctly as you work at your desk, commute through rush-hour traffic, or confront a difficult situation. Breath is life. Become intimate with it and allow it to sustain, nourish, and enhance the quality of your life, moment to moment.

The *Asanas*

Buddhists use the term *beginner's mind.* It means a state of awareness and childlike curiosity that we as adults have lost though the distractions and stress of everyday life. It is a state of being that allows our mind to clear away clutter and eliminate illusion. It brings us into the present, opening a window in our mind that allows the light to illuminate our path.

As we begin each yoga practice, we should approach our mat with a beginner's mind. By taking a moment in Mountain Pose to connect with our breath and center our bodies, we are preparing to enter that state of being in which we are not ruled by our thoughts. Our minds go into neutral while the innate wisdom of our bodies guides us into a deep relationship of wholeness. Our bodies do not lie. By listening, we build the bridge that connects us to our internal world and to the answers that keep us honest, committed, and integrated.

When practiced in this way, each yoga pose, like each day, will be unique. Day to day, practice to practice, you will notice your facility with each pose change. What felt effortless one day may be more difficult the next or vice versa. Each time you practice, no matter the ease or difficulty, you will leave your practice feeling a sense of wholeness and renewal.

There are 31 postures in this practice. Some poses have modifications that should be practiced with props until you feel complete ease in the pose. Never feel that using a prop is cheating. Cheating is forcing your body to do something that it is not ready to do.

Be wise; do what works. If you can't practice every day, commit to three times per week. If you miss a day or a week or a month, don't give up; get back on the mat. You have the right, the power, and the responsibility to live a life of quality and authenticity. The tools to support and enhance your world begin here.

Standing Postures

Standing poses are the foundation of yoga practice. They can include forward and back bending movements, as well as twists. Standing poses are the most beneficial postures for a beginner because they work the large muscles of the legs, hips, and buttocks and help develop strength, stamina, and coordination. All standing postures can and should be modified with yoga props to suit your individual level of fitness.

In keeping with the idea of balance, postures like Mountain Pose (*Tadasana*; see p. 88) and Triangle Pose (*Trikonasana*; see p. 110) teach you to integrate your upper and lower body, to tone and balance your physical being, and to quiet your mind and look inside.

No matter which standing pose you are practicing, the emphasis is the same. Root into your legs by squaring your feet securely on the ground (your weight should be distributed evenly among your heels and your big and little toes, engaging the quadriceps and lifting the kneecaps). Lengthen the spine, shoulders down. Standing poses help to build strength and release tightness. This newly awakened strength and flexibility will create "space" in your body that takes stress off your joints and allows you to breathe more fully. If you practice standing poses regularly, you will develop a more graceful, agile body and a sense of confidence that comes from inner strength.

Forward Bends

Because we bend forward regularly in our daily lives, you may be surprised to learn that of all yoga postures, forward bends are potentially the most dangerous. If practiced incorrectly, they're a lot like forcing your body to reach your toes before it's conditioned to do so. Correct forward bending—from the hips—is most often restricted by hamstring muscles that have become too tight. These muscles, on the back of your thigh, connect to the bone behind the knee and at the sit bones. They are strong, stabilizing muscles and make up one of the largest muscle groups. Tight hamstrings force us to bend from the lower back instead, reversing the natural forward curve of the spine. When we repeatedly bend forward incorrectly, we weaken the muscles that support the back and potentially cause damage to the spine. When practiced correctly, forward bends can help relieve back discomfort by balancing strength and flexibility of the entire back of the body. Forward bends can be done standing or seated and should be modified with a brick or a strap so that correct alignment can be achieved without force or strain. They have a quieting effect on the nervous system and can help to relieve stress and soothe you to sleep.

Twists

In order to achieve a balanced body, we must take time to move in all the directions for which our bodies were intended. The spine bends forward and backward, but it also rotates and bends to the side. Twisting movements are important to help keep mobility in the spine and to tone the smaller muscles that provide structural support, which are often weak and sore from lack of use. Twists can bring relief to the back, neck, and shoulders by relieving tension and stiffness.

In addition to the postural effects, twists have an amazingly powerful effect on your internal organs. When you are doing standing or seated twists, the movement begins from the base of your spine, so the postures involve all of the organs of your torso. As you exhale and twist, you are compressing these organs, which has the effect of "wringing out" or releasing toxins—think of wringing out a sponge. As you inhale and release the twist, the organs can then more readily absorb blood and oxygen, which helps to tone and strengthen them. Twists also aid digestion and elimination, which help to keep the body free of impurities. They have a warming effect on the body and are stimulating to the nervous system.

Back Bends

Try this: Slump forward. Now try to take a deep breath. It's almost impossible. Yet our typical daily routines—driving, sitting at a computer, riding in an airplane—take us into a slumped, rounded-forward position so that the backward curves of the spine become overly rounded. This posture is not only structurally damaging; it also prevents proper breathing by compressing your lungs, and proper digestion by compressing your stomach and intestines.

Over time, you become "locked" in this rounded position because it is the only movement your body knows. Back bends stretch the spinal curves in the opposite direction. They tone and strengthen the muscles that have weakened from lack of use and help to restore a more youthful, graceful carriage. They stretch the chest and abdominal muscles and organs, making space for breath and improved function.

When practicing back bends, exercise caution: The forward curve of the lower back will move into a back bend quite effortlessly, but you can cause compression in this area by bending only where it is easiest. A proper back bend incorporates the entire spinal column evenly.

Back bends are known to free the energy of the spine, and while some poses are quite challenging, they are the most invigorating of all yoga postures.

YOGA SUTRA 2:46...
The physical postures should be steady and comfortable.

Props

Perhaps you think that you are too stiff, too large, or too old to do yoga. Maybe you have tried a few yoga postures and felt too uncomfortable or awkward to continue. Everyone can benefit from yoga practice, no matter your age, weight, or physical condition. It all depends on *how* you practice.

Yoga is about being where you are in each moment, and that means being honest with yourself. You can't go from point A to point E; you must go breath by breath, moment by moment. Forcing your body into a position that it's unfamiliar with or unable to achieve comfortably is dishonest and creates stress.

Yoga props can help you achieve postures that would otherwise be too difficult, and they allow you to experience each pose in correct alignment without overstretching muscles or straining joints. It is important to know that using a yoga prop is not cheating. They were originally designed by B. K. S. Iyengar and are an integral part of his teaching. The use of yoga props can help you balance your strength with your flexibility and allow you to receive the benefits of the each posture with wisdom and integrity.

Mat

A yoga mat has a slightly sticky texture that helps you keep your feet in place when practicing the standing postures. It also provides cushion for joints and insulation from the floor.

Straps

Yoga straps are used as extensions of the arms or legs. For instance, rather than straining to reach your foot with your hands, place a strap around the ball of your foot and hold the strap with your hands. This allows you to fully straighten your knee so that the muscles are stretched evenly from your sit bone to your heel.

Bricks

The yoga bricks are used to add height to the floor. Using bricks in standing postures helps you maintain length through your spine rather than rounding your back to try to reach the floor.

Blanket

In addition to covering up in Relaxation Pose after practice, you can use your yoga blanket in many ways. In the seated postures, it provides cushioning and also adds elevation so that your pelvis is placed in better alignment for the postures. The blanket can also be used to provide support for your head and neck. When placing the blanket under your head, make sure that it is thinly folded and provides just enough support so that your neck is comfortable. When choosing a blanket for yoga practice, choose one that is thin (no more than a couple of inches high) when folded and preferably made of cotton or wool.

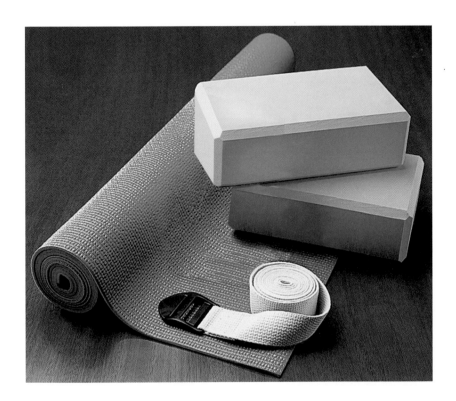

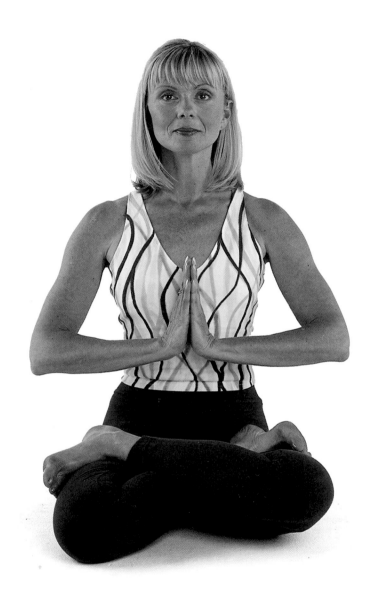

[5]

THE *ASANAS*

Our emotions and physical bodies change day to day. It's important to realize that each time we approach our mat, our levels of strength and flexibility might be different than the time before. Yoga is noncompetitive. It teaches us to listen and respect where we are in each moment. Each time you practice yoga, do so as if you are exploring a new territory. Feel your body with your mind. See with your internal eyes. Listen to the wisdom of your body. Meet your resistances, your strength, and your weaknesses and honor them.

SIMPLE SEATED CROSS LEG
SWASTIKASANA

Let's begin with a few simple yoga postures to warm up the body. Seated poses stretch the hips, thighs, and lower back. The following poses begin with a simple cross-legged seated position, which serves as a base from which we flex and extend the spine. These movements help to gently warm the spinal muscles without requiring too much physical energy.

Benefits

* Stretches the inner thighs and hips

* Relieves stiffness in the lower back

* Creates a seated base from which the spine can extend

Tips

* If you have tight hips, sit on a firmly folded blanket so that your buttocks are raised.

* As you settle into a seated position, shift your weight to your left and pull the flesh of your buttock out from under you toward the back of the mat. Repeat on the other side. This will root the bottom of your pelvis—the part we call the "sit bones"—firmly to the floor and shift it so that your posture is upright.

* Your spine should not be rounded for this pose, so go only as far forward as you can with a long spine.

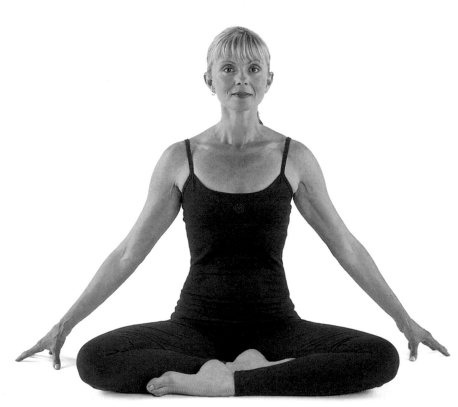

Fig. 1

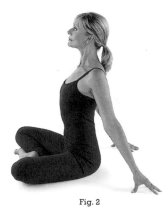

Fig. 2

Fig. 2

✳ Begin in a simple cross-legged position with your right leg folded in first.

✳ Stretch your arms behind you and place your hands on the floor at a comfortable distance, with your fingertips turned away from your body.

✳ Inhale and lift your chest. Pull your shoulder blades down your back as you gently lift your chin.

✳ Breathe for 3 to 5 long, evenly paced breaths.

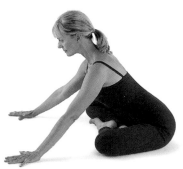

Fig. 3

Fig. 3

✳ With your exhalation, place your hands in front of you. Walk your hands forward until you feel a comfortable stretch in your hips.

✳ Keep your shoulders down and your sit bones on the floor. As you move forward, think of reaching up and out of your pelvis to maintain a lengthened spine.

✳ Breathe for 3 to 5 long, evenly paced breaths.

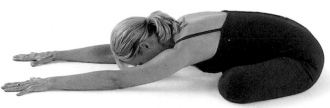

Fig. 4

Fig. 4: Variation

✳ If you have the flexibility, continue to walk your hands forward until you feel a comfortable stretch in your back.

✳ Breathe for 3 to 5 long, evenly paced breaths.

✳ To come out of the pose, use your hands to walk up, inhaling as you do so. Recross your legs with the opposite leg folded in closest to you and repeat for 3 to 5 breaths.

SEATED SPINAL TWIST

Simple cross-legged twists help to stretch and strengthen the muscles that wrap diagonally around the torso. This can help to improve your breathing, tone the waist, and relieve muscular tension.

Benefits

* Keeps the spinal column supple

* Releases tension and fatigue

* Improves posture

* Tones internal organs

Things to remember

* *Breathe.*

* *Twist only as much as you can while maintaining a steady, rhythmic breath.*

* *Do not force the twist.*

* *Lengthen your spine in every movement.*

Tip

* Sit high enough so that your knees are below your waist and your lower back curves slightly forward. Use a blanket if necessary.

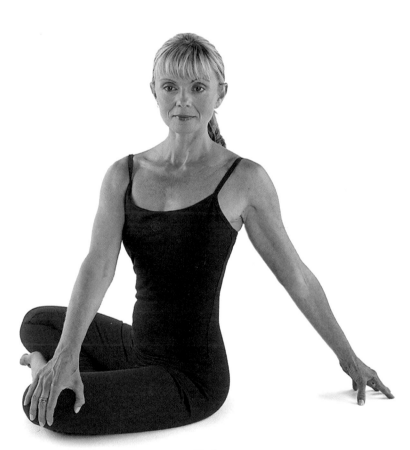

Fig. 1

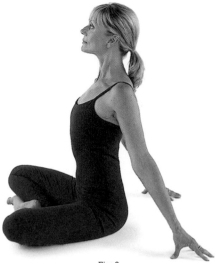

Fig. 2

Fig. 2

⁎ Settle into a proper seated position, as described in the Simple Seated Cross Leg (see p. 78).

⁎ Place your hands a comfortable distance behind you, turning your fingers away from you.

⁎ Inhale and lift your chest.

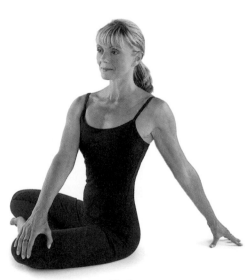

Fig. 3

Fig. 3

⁎ As you exhale, turn your torso to the right, while maintaining a lengthened spine. Place your left hand on your right knee and reach back to rest your right hand behind you.

⁎ Inhale and further lengthen your spine. As you exhale, twist more to your right, moving from your lower abdomen. The twist should originate in your lower torso, not in your shoulders and neck.

⁎ Inhale as you lengthen upward to create space in your spinal column and torso.

⁎ Exhale from your lower abdominals to assist you in the twist.

⁎ Breathe for 3 to 5 long, evenly paced breaths.

⁎ Come back to center, inhale, and exhale as you repeat on the other side.

CAT/COW POSE

MARJARYASANA

These simple poses will help you connect the movement of your body to the flowing rhythm of your breathing. As you exhale and round your spine, use your abdominal muscles to help expel the breath. As you inhale and arch your spine, invite the breath deeply into your lungs. Feel the breath washing through your body like a wave. These movements have a tranquilizing, soothing effect upon the mind and body. They also help to tone the abdomen and keep the spine supple.

Benefits

* Connects you to your breath and the rhythmic movement of your body

* Stretches and tones the spine

* Helps develop coordination

* Tones the hips, butt, and thighs

* Develops shoulder strength

* Stretches the wrists

Things to remember

* *Keep your abdominals engaged to assist your movement and to protect your lower back.*

* *Feel your body as you move and breathe.*

* *Press through your arms and hands evenly to assist your balance.*

* *Keep your shoulder blades spread wide and moving down your back.*

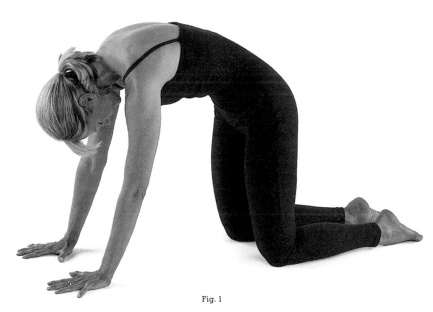

Fig. 1

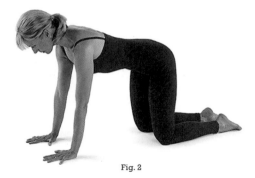

Fig. 2

Fig. 2

＊ Begin on all fours with your hands under your shoulders and knees under your hips. Your spine should be in a neutral position.

＊ Inhale to lengthen your spine.

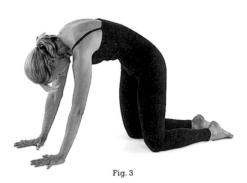

Fig. 3

Fig. 3

＊ As you exhale, pull your abdominals in, curl your tailbone to the floor, lift your rib cage to the ceiling, and release your neck to bow your head.

＊ Keep your shoulder blades wide and feel them moving down your back. This is Cat Pose.

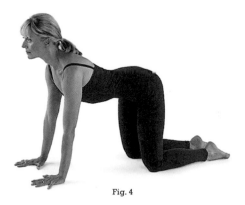

Fig. 4

Fig. 4

＊ From Cat Pose, inhale and lift your tailbone as you roll through your spine to extend your chest forward, shoulders down. Lift your chin slightly and look straight ahead. This is Cow Pose.

＊ Using your breath to help you move, exhale and pull your abdominals in, rounding your spine to come back into Cat Pose. Alternate between the two positions 3 to 5 times.

＊ Inhale and come to a neutral spine.

CAT/COW POSE WITH LEG EXTENSIONS

MARJARYASANA WITH LEG EXTENSIONS

Incorporating the leg extension into Cat/Cow Pose requires more coordination and balance. Do this movement slowly and precisely. As you extend your leg, imagine lengthening through your torso and out the crown of your head, and simultaneously through your leg and out through your toes. Keep your abdominal muscles engaged to support your torso in the lengthened position and use them to help expel the breath in the tucked position. Your breath should be in harmony with the movement of your body.

Benefits

* Develops balance and coordination

* Tones hips, thighs, buttocks, and waist

* Teaches stillness and movement simultaneously

Things to remember

* *As your leg extends back, support your center with your abdominal muscles.*

* *Move slowly, with the rhythm of your breath.*

* *Press through your arms; keep your shoulder blades and upper back wide.*

Tip

* As you move, imagine your spine moving in a straight line from your tailbone through the top of your head. Don't let yourself sway from side to side; control the movement.

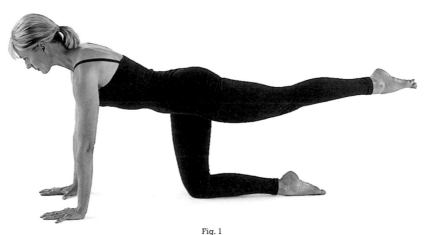

Fig. 1

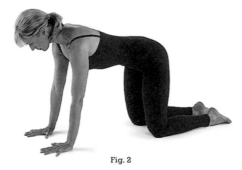

Fig. 2

Fig. 2

✳ From Cat/Cow Pose (see p. 72), inhale and come to a neutral spine.

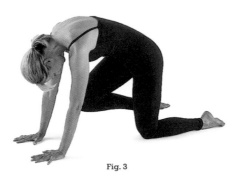

Fig. 3

Fig. 3

✳ Exhale and pull your abdominals in as you curl your tailbone toward the mat, widen your upper back, and tuck your right knee toward your chest.

✳ Relax your neck and release your head.

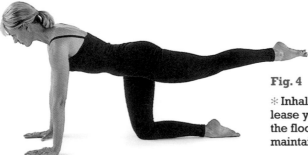

Fig. 4

Fig. 4

✳ Inhale as you extend your right leg behind you. Release your chin from your chest and look directly at the floor, so that your neck is lengthened. Try to maintain a steady balance as you do this.

✳ Keep your body strong and lengthen from your extended toes through the top of your head.

✳ Repeat the movement three to five times with each leg. Use the rhythm of your breath to control your movements.

✳ Change sides and repeat with the opposite leg.

CHILD'S POSE
BALASANA

Child's Pose replicates the position where life begins in the womb. It has a very soothing effect on the nervous system because it stretches the spinal column. This position increases the awareness of feeling the breath in your back, helping you to breathe more deeply. This gentle stretch is also very safe for the lower back because your body is supported over your legs and there is little chance of overstretching. Child's Pose is also used as a rest position during a long sequence of *asanas.*

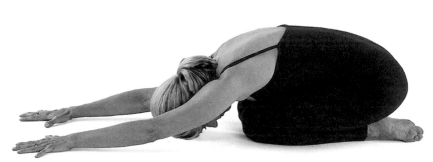

Fig. 1

Benefits

* Gently stretches the back and shoulders

* Soothes the mind and quiets the nervous system

Things to remember

* *Breathe.*

* *Use support to rest your forehead.*

* *Place your arms in the most comfortable position.*

Tips

* If you experience discomfort in your ankles or knees, place a small rolled towel or washcloth under your ankles or behind your knees to relieve pressure.

* Choose the less demanding modification if discomfort continues.

* The pressure of the brick or the floor against your forehead is soothing to the mind and can help relieve headaches.

* Resting your arms at your sides is a more soothing way to do this pose.

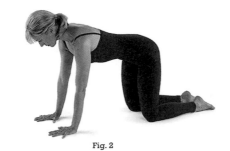

Fig. 2

Fig. 2

✳ Begin on your hands and knees with your hands under your shoulders and your knees under your hips. Inhale to lengthen your spine.

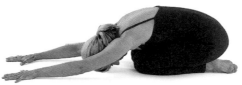

Fig. 3

Fig. 3

✳ Exhale as you move your hips back and sit on your heels. Allow your body to be supported by your thighs.

✳ Stretching your arms forward helps to open tight shoulders.

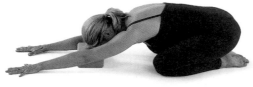

Fig. 4

Fig. 4: *Modification*

✳ If the full pose is uncomfortable, from your hands and knees, separate your knees and move your hips back to sit on your heels. Rest your head on a brick and stretch your arms forward.

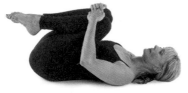

Fig. 5

Fig. 5: *Variation*

✳ Lie on your back. One at a time, bring your knees to your chest. Wrap your arms around your knees and pull them gently toward your chest.

MOUNTAIN POSE (WITH BREATH)
TADASANA

Rooting the legs to the earth while moving the arms through space and breathing rhythmically helps the body and the mind understand how to move and be still simultaneously. This is a wonderful flowing pose to do in the morning to calm and balance your energy.

Benefits

* Teaches stillness and movement simultaneously

* Promotes postural awareness and helps to correct imbalances

* Improves balance and coordination

* Quiets the mind; helps to integrate mind and body

Things to remember

* *Keep your weight balanced on the four corners of your feet.*

* *Do not lock your knee joints.*

* *Move your legs and feet downward into the earth; lengthen your spine upward though the top of your head.*

* *Maintain the lower-rib-to-hipbone connection as your arms come overhead.*

* *Keep your shoulders down and your elbows straight as you reach overhead.*

* *Move as though the rhythm of your breath were making the movement happen.*

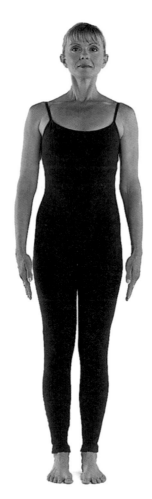

Fig. 1

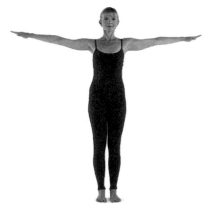

Fig. 2

Fig. 2

＊ Begin with your feet hip-width apart and parallel. Your heels should be under your sit bones. Spread your toes wide and feel grounded in your stance. This is Mountain Pose.

＊ Inhale and raise your arms out to your sides.

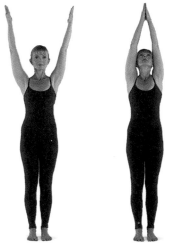

Fig. 3   Fig. 4

Figs. 3 and 4

＊ Turn your palms up and reach overhead.

＊ If you can, bring your palms together overhead; look toward your hands.

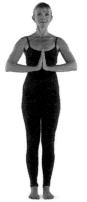

Fig. 5

Fig. 5

＊ Exhale and lower your arms to your sides. Bring your palms together in front of your heart in *namaste,* or Prayer Pose.

＊ Repeat these movements for 5 to 10 breaths, inhaling as you raise your arms and exhaling as they release to your sides.

＊ After your final repetition, pause with palms together in *namaste.* Close your eyes and feel your body in space. Align yourself once again from the soles of your feet upward.

CHAIR POSE
UTKATASANA

Chair Pose focuses attention on the lower body. When the ankles and hips are flexed and the knees bent, the muscles of the legs, hips, and buttocks are challenged to support the weight of the body. Because the upper body is angled forward, the abdominal muscles must engage to protect the lower back. This effort strengthens, tones, and sculpts all of the acting muscle groups. Gradually raising the arms helps to increase flexibility in the shoulders and relieve upper back tension.

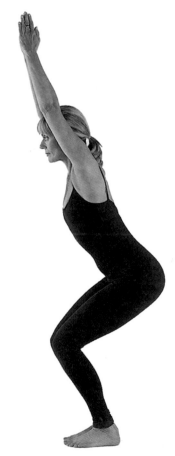

Fig. 1

Benefits

* Teaches balance, coordination, and stamina

* Strengthens ankles, calves, and thighs

* Stretches and tones the abdominal muscles and organs

* Opens the chest for improved breathing

Things to remember

* *Bring your feet together if comfortable.*

* *Keep your shoulders down and elbows straight as you reach your arms overhead.*

* *Feel the connection between your lower ribs and hipbones. (In Chair Pose, it's particularly important not to arch your lower back.)*

* *Keep the back of your neck long.*

* *Stand evenly on both feet, keeping your weight on your heels and the balls of your feet.*

* *Your eyes should maintain a soft forward gaze; forehead and temples stay relaxed.*

* *Don't hold your breath!*

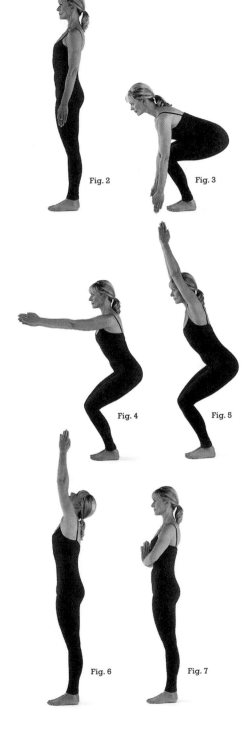

Fig. 2

Fig. 3

Fig. 4

Fig. 5

Fig. 6

Fig. 7

Figs. 2 and 3

＊ Begin in Mountain Pose (see p. 88), heels under your sit bones.

＊ Exhale and bend your knees. Shift your hips back as if sitting in a chair.

Figs. 4 and 5

＊ Inhale, raise your torso, and stretch your arms straight forward from the shoulder. Keep your shoulders down. Spread your toes and press into the balls of your feet. Keep your lower-rib-to-hipbone connection. Exhale.

＊ Stretch your arms overhead and bring your hands together until your palms touch. Keep your elbows straight.

＊ Breathe for 5 to 10 evenly paced breaths.

Figs. 6 and 7

＊ Reaching upward, inhale and straighten your legs.

＊ Exhale, lowering your arms to your sides; then bring your palms together in front of your heart in *namaste*.

＊ Repeat twice, exhaling as you bend your knees and inhaling as you raise your arms and straighten your legs.

TWISTING CHAIR POSE
TWISTING UTKATASANA

Twisting Chair Pose is a variation of the classic Chair Pose. Strength that is developed in Chair Pose can be challenged by twisting the upper body to the right and left. This requires balance, coordination, and flexibility. Twisting the torso helps to stimulate digestion and elimination, while warming and toning the internal organs.

Benefits

* Teaches stability, balance, coordination, and stamina

* Strengthens ankles, calves, and thighs

* Stretches and tones muscles of the abdomen, waist, and sides

* Stimulates internal organs

Things to remember

* Hips, knees, and ankles should remain still while you twist.

* Keep your shoulders down away from your ears.

* Maintain your rib-to-hipbone connection.

* Turn your torso, not your head, and keep your nose in line with your breastbone.

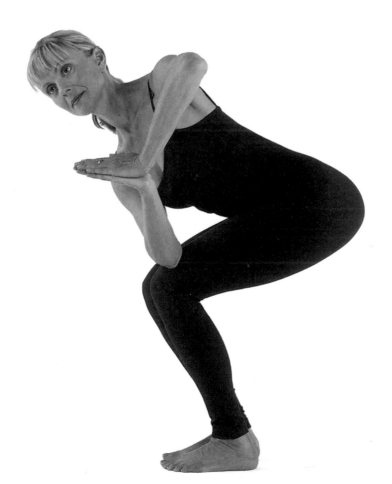

Fig. 1

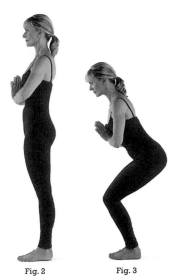

Fig. 2   Fig. 3

Figs. 2 and 3

❋ Begin in Mountain Pose (see p. 88), with your hands in *namaste*.

❋ Exhale and bend your knees, lowering yourself into Chair Pose (see p. 90).

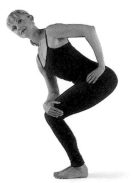

Fig. 4

Fig. 4

❋ Inhale. As you exhale, twist your torso to the right, keeping your pelvis still as you do so.

❋ Place your left hand on your right knee and your right hand on your right outer hip.

❋ Breathe for 5 to 10 evenly paced breaths.

❋ Exhale and return your torso and arms to center. Inhale, straighten your legs, and stretch your arms up; then exhale and return your hands to *namaste*. Repeat on the other side.

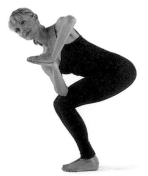

Fig. 5

Fig. 5

❋ Exhale and bend your knees, lowering yourself into Chair Pose.

❋ Inhale. As you exhale, bring your hands into *namaste* and, keeping your pelvis still, twist your torso to the right. Cross your left elbow over your right knee. Keep your palms in front of your heart in Prayer Pose and your chin in line with your breastbone.

❋ Breathe for 5 to 10 evenly paced breaths.

❋ Inhale and straighten your legs, stretching your arms up, then exhale and return your hands to *namaste*. Repeat on the other side.

STANDING FORWARD BEND
UTTANASANA

Practice this pose to calm and restore your energy during a stressful day. Nerve impulses run between the body and the mind through the spinal column. Stretching the spine has a profound effect upon our ability to calm down and relieve tension from our bodies and stress from our minds. Standing Forward Bend is a favorite pose of many yoga students because it feels great and can be done just about anywhere. The next time you are on a plane or sitting at your computer for long periods, try this pose every few minutes to relieve and refresh your mind and body.

Benefits

* Releases tension from the legs, hips, and lower back by teaching proper stretching of the hamstrings

* Stretches the spine

* Helps relieve abdominal pain during menstruation

* Slows the heart rate

* Calms the mind

* Stretches and rejuvenates the spinal nerves

Things to remember

* *Provide proper support, using a brick if necessary.*

* *Stretch your hamstring muscles fully before attempting to stretch your back.*

* *Never push to discomfort or compromised breath.*

* *Distribute your weight evenly on the four corners of the feet.*

* *Straighten your legs without locking your knees.*

* *Stay mindful of your breathing.*

* *As you begin to feel comfortable and stable in this pose, try doing it with your feet closer together.*

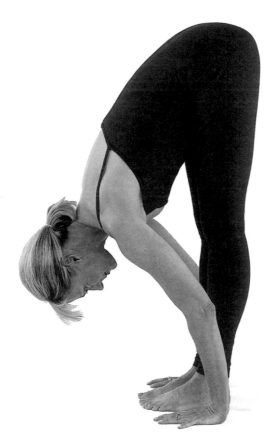

Fig. 1

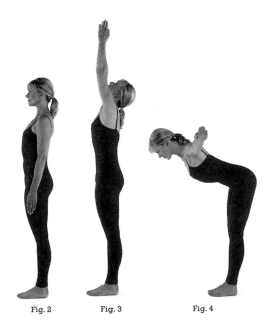

Fig. 2

Fig. 2

* Begin in Mountain Pose (see p. 88), arms at your sides.

Fig. 3

* Inhale and bring your arms out to the sides and overhead, palms facing each other.

Fig. 4

* Exhale as you release your arms to your sides, and then fold forward from your hips. Use your abdominal muscles for support.

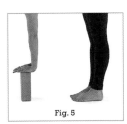

Fig. 5

Fig. 5: Modification

* Lower your arms and place your hands on a brick for support. The brick should be under your nose. You may use the brick in the high (vertical), medium (horizontal and on its side), or low (horizontal and flat) position.

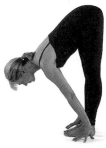

Fig. 6

Fig. 6

* As you become more flexible, you may place your hands on the floor outside your feet.

* Elongate your spine and fold deeply from your hips. If you feel strain in your back, continue to use the brick. Press the heels of your hands to the mat or brick.

* Breathe for 5 to 10 evenly paced breaths.

* Inhale and simultaneously raise your upper body from the floor, keeping your spine long, and bring your out arms to the sides and overhead. Your arms should arrive overhead when you have returned to a standing position.

* Exhale and release your arms, bringing your hands to *namaste*.

LUNGE

You may have seen athletes preparing for an event with a variation of this dynamic pose. In a yoga lunge, the body is precisely aligned so that a balance of strength and flexibility is developed in the lower body and the joints are protected from strain. It is important to read the directions carefully and stand up in the full pose only when you are strong, stable, and breathing easily in one of the modifications. The use of a brick can be helpful if you have flexibility issues.

Benefits

* Stretches, tones, and balances the muscles of the lower body to prepare for standing postures

* Teaches balance in an asymmetrical position

* Improves coordination

* Builds stamina

Things to remember

* *Keep your forward shin vertical to protect your knee joint.*

* *Keep your shoulders down and lengthen through your back leg.*

* *Balance the weight of your pelvis between the strength of your two legs.*

* *Press down though your forward heel to help keep your body lifted.*

* *Support should come from your legs, not your arms.*

Tip

* Use this posture in combination with the Standing Forward Bend (p. 94) and Wide-Leg Standing Forward Bend (p. 98) as a great warm-up and cooldown for other activities, such as walking, running, and biking.

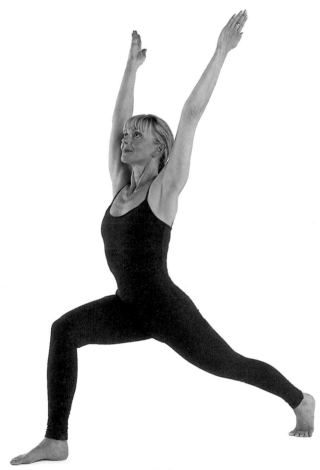

Fig. 1

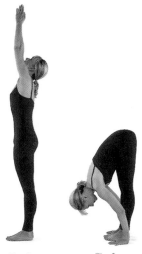

Fig. 2

Fig. 3

Figs. 2 and 3

✳ Begin in Mountain Pose (see p. 88), stretching your arms overhead. Exhale and fold forward from your hips, placing your hands on bricks—or on the mat if you can reach the floor.

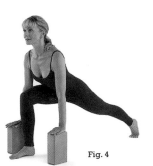

Fig. 4

Fig. 4

✳ Use bricks to modify this pose.

Fig. 5

✳ Inhale, and as you exhale, step your right foot back about 3 feet. The shin of your left leg should be vertical.

✳ Keep the toes of your back foot turned under as you lengthen your back leg and your spine in opposition.

✳ Press down into your forward foot, feeling about two-thirds of your weight in your heel.

✳ Lengthen out through your back leg.

✳ Breathe for 5 to 10 long, evenly paced breaths.

✳ Press into your forward heel, spring off your back toes, and step to a Standing Forward Bend (see p. 94). Step back with your left leg and repeat the pose on the other side.

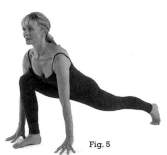

Fig. 5

✳ Release back to Standing Forward Bend. Inhale, raise your upper body, and bring your arms to the sides and overhead. Exhale and release your arms, bringing your hands to *namaste.*

Option for full pose

✳ From low lunge position, inhale and bring your arms to your sides and overhead.

✳ Press down through your forward heel and lengthen out through your back leg.

✳ Lift your rib cage off your waist as you lengthen your side body into your arms.

✳ Breathe for 5 to 10 long, evenly paced breaths.

✳ Exhale and release your hands to the mat or bricks.

WIDE-LEG STANDING FORWARD BEND
PRASARITA PADOTTANASANA

Some people find this pose more comfortable than the classic Standing Forward Bend. Because the feet are wide and the legs are at an angle to the hip socket, however, more stability is required from the legs, ankles, and feet to maintain correct alignment. When practiced properly, this posture can have a powerful effect on toning and sculpting the legs, strengthening the ankles and the feet, and relieving tension and stress. Folding forward also increases blood flow to the torso, which aids digestion.

Benefits

* Stretches and tones the ankles and calves and inner and outer thighs

* Aids digestion

* Relieves tension in the hips and lower back

Things to remember

* *Ankles have a tendency to roll outward in this pose. Press through the inner edge of your feet to balance the weight on the four corners of your feet.*

* *Provide proper support, using a brick if needed. Never overstretch.*

* *Breathe.*

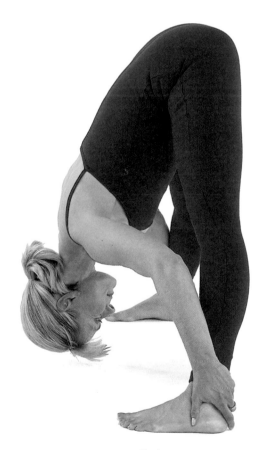

Fig. 1

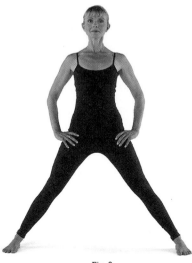

Fig. 2

Fig. 2

✳ Begin by stepping your feet 3 to 4 feet apart. The outer edges of your feet should be parallel to the outer edges of the mat.

✳ Place your hands at your hip creases (where your legs and hips meet).

✳ Plant your legs firmly and distribute your weight evenly across your feet, spreading your toes.

✳ Inhale and lengthen your spine upward, lifting your chest.

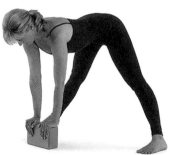

Fig. 3

Fig. 3

✳ Exhale and fold forward from your hip creases, allowing your pelvis to tip forward. Place your hands on a brick or the floor.

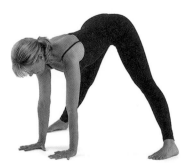

Fig. 4

Fig. 4

✳ Distribute your weight evenly across the four corners of your feet. Firm the front of your legs so that your kneecaps lift and point forward in line with your middle toes.

✳ Breathe for 5 to 10 evenly paced breaths.

✳ Or, you can fold even more deeply and hold the outsides of your ankles (see Fig. 1).

✳ Inhale and come up with a long spine.

WIDE-LEG DOWNWARD-FACING DOG POSE

This is a wide-leg variation of the classic Downward-Facing Dog Pose (see p. 112). When the feet are separated wider than the hips, the pelvis has greater ability to properly tip forward from the hip creases. This allows more length in the spine and through the shoulders. It also creates a wider base for a greater sense of balance and stability.

Benefits

* Calms the mind

* Stretches and tones the legs

* Brings circulation to the torso to aid digestion

* Stretches shoulders and releases tension

Things to remember

* *Keep your legs strong, your kneecaps lifted and pointed forward, and your weight distributed evenly across your feet.*

* *Keep your arms strong as if pushing the floor away from you.*

* *Keep your shoulder blades wide and feel them moving down your back to avoid neck tension.*

* *Keep your abdominal muscles firm to support your center.*

* *Think of moving your weight up and back off your hands and into your feet.*

* *Breathe evenly.*

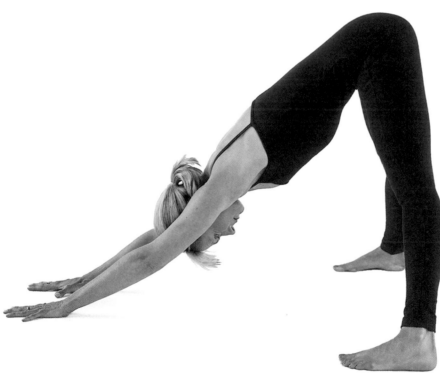

Fig. 1

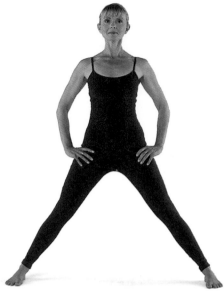

Fig. 2

Fig. 2

✳ Begin with your feet 3 to 4 feet apart. The outer edges of your feet should be parallel to the outer edges of your mat.

✳ Place your hands at your hip creases (where your legs and hips meet) and press down.

✳ Plant your legs firmly and distribute your weight evenly across your feet, spreading your toes.

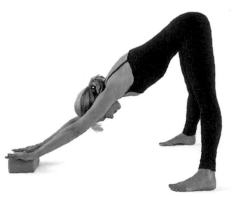

Fig. 3

Fig. 3

✳ Inhale, then exhale, folding forward from your hip creases and allowing your pelvis to tip forward.

✳ Place your hands on a brick in front of you. Lengthen through your spine and press down through your heels.

✳ Breathe for 5 to 10 long, evenly paced breaths.

✳ Inhale to come up, maintaining a long spine.

Option for full pose

✳ If you have the flexibility, place your hands on the floor (see Fig. 1).

SINGLE-LEG STANDING FORWARD BEND

PARSVOTTANASANA

In this series, Single-Leg Standing Forward Bend is the first of the forward bending poses that requires taking the feet into an asymmetrical stance. This stance develops strength and flexibility and helps to improve balance. The position of the arms behind the back opens and stretches the chest, while moving the shoulder blades down helps to tone the midback and improve posture. While you are in the posture, you should keep your breath strong and steady so that the compressed abdominal organs can receive a massage.

Benefits

* Relieves tension in hips and legs

* Helps free the spine for greater mobility

* Stretches the chest for better breathing

* Relieves tension in the shoulders

* Helps correct a slumped posture

Things to remember

* *Balance your weight evenly between your legs; keep your back leg rooted to the earth.*

* *Keep both hip-bones in the same plane, working to move the back hip forward.*

* *Keep the legs and feet rooted into the earth.*

* *Lengthen the spine forward and keep your shoulders pulling down away from your ears.*

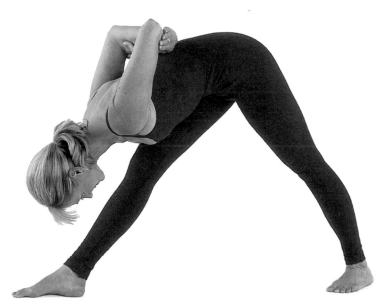

Fig. 1

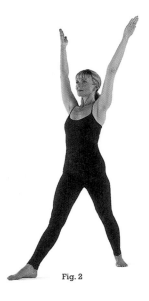

Fig. 2

Fig. 2

❊ Stand in Mountain Pose (see p. 88), with your feet about hip-width apart, and step back about 3 feet with your left foot. Your right foot should be pointing forward in line with your kneecap and hip socket. Your left foot should be turned out at a 45-degree angle and in line with your left hip.

❊ Inhale and bring your arms overhead, palms facing each other. Bring your left hipbone forward to level your pelvis.

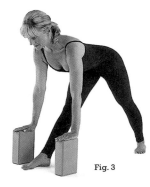

Fig. 3

Fig. 3

❊ Exhale and fold forward from your hips, placing your hands on bricks. Stretch your chest forward from the base of your spine. Keep your lower-rib-to-hipbone connection.

❊ Breathe for 5 to 10 evenly paced breaths.

❊ Inhale and come up. Raise your arms overhead.

❊ Change legs by stepping your right foot back and repeat for 5 to 10 evenly paced breaths on the other side.

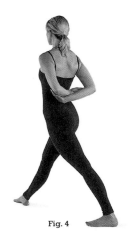

Fig. 4

Fig. 4: *Option for full pose*

❊ Inhale and come up. Bring your arms to shoulder height and exhale, turning your thumbs toward the floor. Bring your arms behind your back and catch hold of your elbows with opposite hands.

❊ Inhale, lifting your chest as you move your shoulder blades down your back.

❊ Exhale and fold forward from your hip creases, allowing your pelvis to tip forward. Keep your hips level. Pull your shoulder blades down, lift your elbows, and stretch your chest forward over your legs (see Fig. 1).

❊ Breathe for 5 to 10 long, evenly paced breaths.

❊ Inhale and come up. Change legs by stepping your right foot back and repeat for 5 to 10 evenly paced breaths on the other side.

❊ Step your feet together into Mountain Pose and bring your hands to *namaste*.

WARRIOR I POSE
VIRABHRDRASANA I

This is the first of the Warrior poses. As its name suggests, it is a strong, full-body pose that requires your full attention to alignment and breathing. The center of the pose is the pelvis, and its placement is important to the correct alignment of the legs and the spine. Because the legs are in an asymmetrical stance, the hip joint of the back leg has a tendency to twist backward. You will have to work to bring the hip joints into alignment. The spine is extended or in a back bend position, so you will have to keep your chest lifted to avoid compressing your lower back.

Things to remember

* *The difference between the modified version and the full pose is the ability to sink deeply into your hips while maintaining the strength of the back leg and the length of the spine.*

* *If you feel compression in your lower back, bend your front knee less, use your abdominals more, and lengthen your tailbone downward.*

* *Do not force your hip forward; breathe and allow your body to gain flexibility and strength with time.*

* *Don't force any one aspect of instruction. Think of your body as a whole and work to achieve a posture in which you can breathe evenly and feel balanced.*

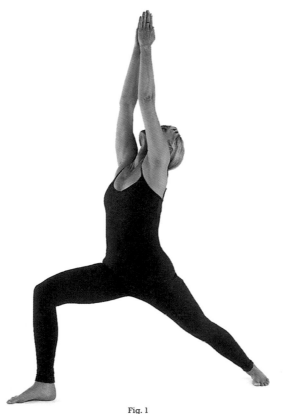

Fig. 1

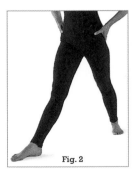

Fig. 2

Fig. 2

✳ Begin in Mountain Pose (see p. 88) and step back about 3 to 4 feet with your left foot. Your feet should be spaced about as wide as your hips and your right foot should be pointing forward in line with your kneecap and hip socket. Your left foot should be turned out at a 45-degree angle and in line with your left hip.

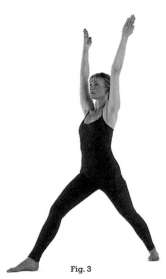

Fig. 3

Fig. 3

✳ Inhale and bring your arms overhead. Exhale and bend your right knee while keeping your left leg strongly rooted to the earth.

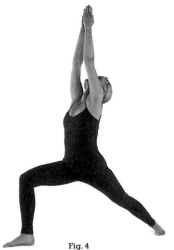

Fig. 4

Fig. 4

✳ Bend your right knee to a right angle over your ankle.

✳ Strongly lift your chest and reach through your arms as you look up to your hands.

✳ Keep your left leg strongly rooted to the earth.

✳ With each breath, think of moving your left hip forward into the same plane with your right hip.

✳ Use your abdominal muscles to support your lower back and lengthen your tailbone downward.

✳ Breathe for 5 to 10 long, evenly paced breaths.

✳ Inhale and straighten your front leg. Step your left foot forward as you exhale, coming back to Mountain Pose. Change legs and hold for 5 to 10 breaths on the other side.

WARRIOR II POSE
VIRABHRDRASANA II

Warrior II Pose is a strong, heat-building posture that develops strength, endurance, and discipline in the body and the mind. As in all yoga postures, the center of the pose is the pelvis, which maintains its neutral position as the forward knee is bent. The spine extends upward into the lift of the chest as the arms reach from the core of the body. The breath is expanded into the entire torso, back and front.

Benefits

* Develops strength and stamina

* Conducts body heat; increases heart rate

* Strengthens legs, hips, and ankles

* Tones abdominal organs

* Strengthens and tones shoulder muscles

Things to remember

* *Press into your forward heel and distribute your weight over the four corners of the foot.*

* *Keep your back leg rooted to the earth, with the four corners of the foot bearing weight evenly.*

* *Lengthen your spine upward from your pelvis.*

* *Keep your pelvis level. Do not lean toward your bent knee.*

* *Keep your shoulders down; hold your arms up as if the sides of your body supported them.*

Tip

* To prevent knee strain, keep your ankle, knee, and hip in alignment.

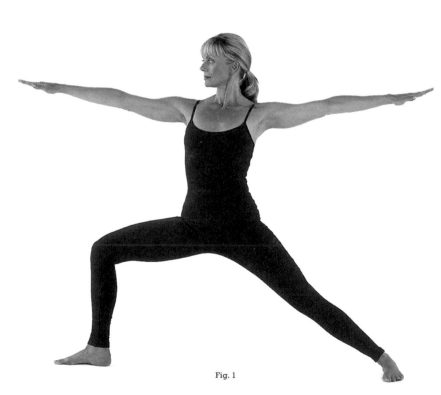

Fig. 1

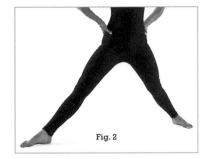

Fig. 2

Fig. 2

* Begin in Mountain Pose (see p. 88) and step your feet about 3 to 4 feet apart.

* Turn your right foot and knee outward from the top of your thigh. Your middle toe, ankle, kneecap, and center hip should be in a straight line.

* Turn your left foot in at a 45-degree angle.

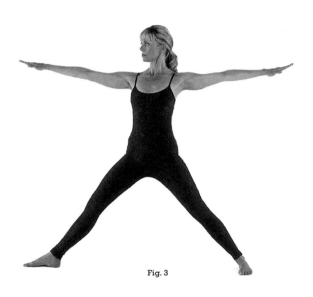

Fig. 3

Fig. 3

* Raise your arms to shoulder height, keeping your shoulders down, your spine extended, and your legs strong.

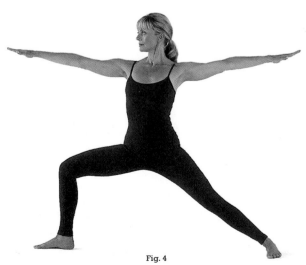

Fig. 4

Fig. 4

* Bend your right knee at a 90-degree angle, centering it over your middle toe. Keep your hipbones level, your spine long, and your weight evenly distributed between your legs.

* Breathe for 5 to 10 evenly paced breaths.

* Inhale and straighten your right leg.

* Turn your left toes out and your right toes in and repeat the pose on the opposite side. Hold for 5 to 10 evenly paced breaths.

* Step your feet together into Mountain Pose, bringing your palms to *namaste.*

EXTENDED SIDE STRETCH
PARSVOKONASANA

This is one of my personal favorites! Extended Side Stretch tones the ankles, knees, and thighs and also helps to shape the hips and buttocks. The side-bending movement of the spine helps to stretch and trim the waist. It also improves breathing by stretching the muscles around the rib cage. The compression of the lower abdomen aids digestion and elimination.

Benefits

* Tones and shapes the ankles, calves, and thighs

* Aids digestion

* Helps trim and tone the waist

* Relieves tension in the spine

Things to remember

* *Keep the front shin vertical.*

* *Press into your forward heel to help activate and balance the muscles of your legs.*

* *Distribute your weight evenly between your legs.*

* *Feel the stretch in the inner thighs and outer hips.*

* *Continue reaching through the back leg to gain more length from the spine.*

* *Use enough support so that you can breathe evenly.*

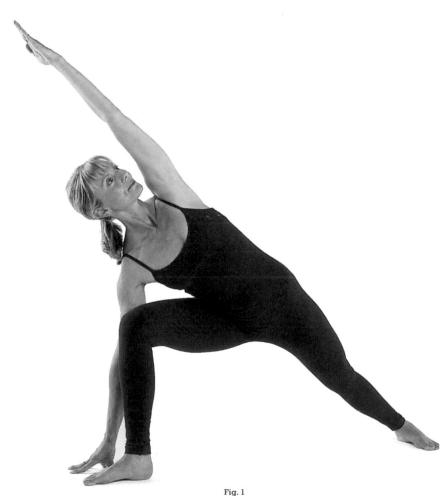

Fig. 1

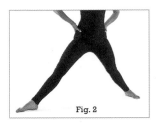

Fig. 2

Fig. 2

* Begin by separating your feet 3 to 4 feet.

* Turn your right foot and knee outward from the top of your thigh.

* Turn your left foot in at a 45-degree angle.

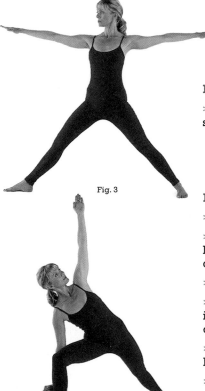

Fig. 3

Fig. 3

* Inhale and raise your arms to shoulder height, keeping your shoulders down, your spine extended, and your legs strong.

Fig. 4

Fig. 4

* Exhale and bend your right knee over your middle toe.

* Lengthen the right side of your waist as you place your right hand on a brick that's at an appropriate height for comfort and correct alignment.

* Extend your top arm straight up.

* Press your forward heel into the mat, press your forward knee into your arm, and fully extend your back leg as you root the four corners of your feet into the mat.

* Lengthen and rotate your spine as you look toward your top hand.

* Breathe for 5 to 10 long, evenly paced breaths.

* Inhale and straighten your right leg to come up. Turn your left toes out and your right toes in at a 45-degree angle. Repeat the pose on the other side.

Option for full pose

* Lengthen your waist as you reach your finger-tips or palm to the mat (see Fig. 1).

* Press into your forward heel and balance your weight across the four corners of your foot.

* Lengthen into your back leg and stretch your spine in opposition.

* Lengthen and rotate your spine as you extend your arm and look toward your left upper arm as you reach it along your ear and over your head (see Fig. 1).

* Breathe for 5 to 10 evenly paced breaths.

* Step your feet together into Mountain Pose, bringing your hands into *namaste.*

TRIANGLE POSE

TRIKONASANA

Triangle pose is one of the more complicated poses to learn without having a teacher to guide your body into the correct alignment. This simple test will let you know if you are moving in the right direction: Stand with your back against a wall. Turn your right foot out and your left foot in. Raise your arms to shoulder height. Exhale and move your hips to the left as you lengthen your torso to the right. Once there, continue to lengthen your spine from the tailbone to the top of your head. When the spine is lengthened fully, rotate your chest upward so that your left shoulder blade moves toward the wall. Keep both sides of your waist long and use your breath to deepen your pose rather than your will or ego.

Benefits

* Strengthens and tones the legs, hips, and abdomen

* Relieves stiffness in the spine

Things to remember

* *If you experience discomfort in your forward knee, take care to rotate your entire leg outward from the upper thigh. Firm the outer hip and lengthen the inner thigh.*

* *Use a brick to avoid strain.*

* *Keep your back leg firmly rooted to help lengthen your spine.*

Tip

* If your neck bothers you while in this pose, look at the floor or straight in front of you.

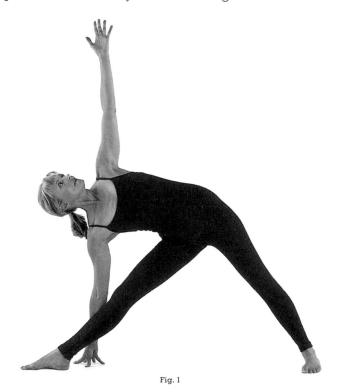

Fig. 1

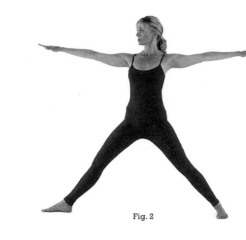

Fig. 2

Fig. 2

* Begin in Mountain Pose (see p. 88) and step your feet 3 to 4 feet apart.

* Turn your right foot and knee outward from the top of your thigh.

* Turn your left foot in at a 45-degree angle amd distribute your weight evenly between your legs.

* Inhale and raise your arms to shoulder height. Keep your shoulders down and stretch out from your core into your fingertips.

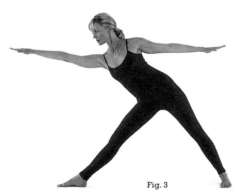

Fig. 3

Fig. 3

* Exhale and extend your side body out over your right leg as you move your hips toward your back foot.

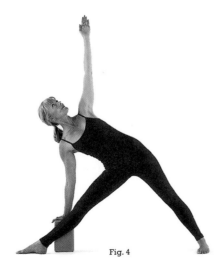

Fig. 4

Fig. 4

* Place your right hand on a brick in the high, medium, or low position. Keep your back leg strongly rooted to the earth. Straighten your left arm overhead and look toward your left hand.

* Breathe for 5 to 10 long, evenly paced breaths.

* Inhale and come up. Turn your left toes out and your right foot in at a 45-degree angle. Repeat the pose on the other side.

* Inhale and come up. Step into Mountain Pose; bring your hands to *namaste.*

Option for full pose

* Place your fingertips on the mat. Keep both sides of your waist long, your chest lifted, and your legs strong (see Fig. 1).

* Breathe for 5 to 10 evenly paced breaths.

DOWNWARD-FACING DOG POSE

ADHO MUKA SVANASANA

If you have time to do only one yoga pose, do Downward-Facing Dog. It stretches and tones the legs and abdominals, lifts the diaphragm for easy breathing, slows the heart rate to calm the mind, relieves tension from the back and shoulders, and invigorates your entire being. Puppy Pose is a variation of the pose that prepares the upper body for the full pose by stretching the shoulders and opening the chest.

Benefits

* Effectively stretches the entire body
* Calms the nervous system
* Strengthens legs and abdominal muscles
* Relieves shoulder tension
* Invigorates
* Relieves stress

Things to remember

* *Distribute your weight on your hands evenly through the roots of the fingers and the heels of the hands. Make sure your middle finger is pointing forward.*

* *Keep your shoulder blades separated.*

* *Do not push your chest to the mat. Instead, it should feel as if your hips are pulling the weight off your hands and back into your heels.*

* *Maintain your lower-rib-to-hipbone connection.*

* *Pull the front of your thighs back and press into your heels.*

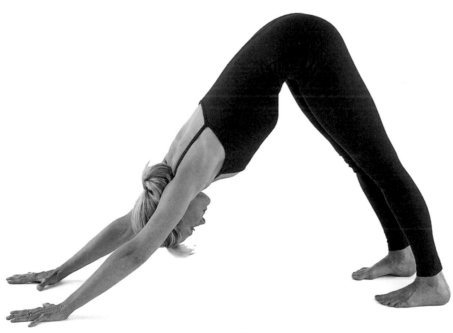

Fig. 1

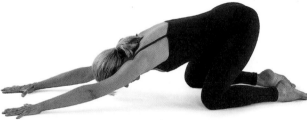

Fig. 2

Fig. 2

In preparation for Dog Pose, use Puppy Pose:

* Start on all fours, placing your hands under your shoulders and your knees under your hips. Walk your knees back 6 to 8 inches.

* Inhale, and as you exhale, keep your arms straight and slide your hips backward. Your hips should end up above your knees, with your spine long and shoulders stretched.

* Breathe for 5 to 10 evenly paced breaths. Inhale as you come up.

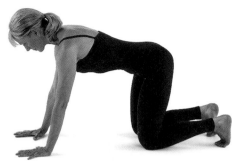

Fig. 3

Fig. 3

* Again on all fours, place your hands directly under your shoulders, spreading your fingers wide.

* Place your knees directly under your hips and turn your toes under.

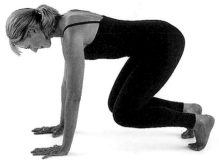

Fig. 4

Fig. 4

* Press through your arms, lift your knees, and move your hips back in space.

* Pressing your sit bones up to the ceiling, pull your thighs back to straighten your legs and press your heels to the mat (see Fig. 1).

* Breathe for 5 to 10 long, evenly paced breaths.

* Exhale, bend your knees, and come to rest in Child's Pose (see p. 86).

HERO'S POSE
VIRASANA

Hero's Pose stretches the muscles in the front of the thighs, lower legs, and ankles and feet. The position of the arms overhead and behind the back helps to relieve tension in the shoulders and upper back and opens the chest for better breathing.

Benefits

* Opens shoulders and chest

* Lengthens sides of body

* Stretches wrists

* Stretches thighs and ankles

Things to remember

* *Use enough support to prevent knee strain.*

* *Keep your lower-rib-to-hipbone connection.*

* *Do not roll your ankles or turn your feet inward or outward.*

* *Sit evenly on your sit bones.*

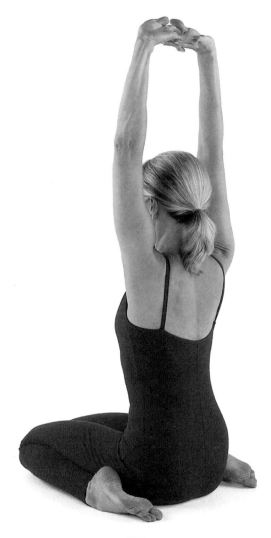

Fig. 1

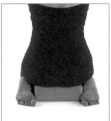

Fig. 2

Fig. 2

* Begin on your hands and knees. Place the tops of your feet on the mat and place a brick between your ankles. Sit back on the brick.

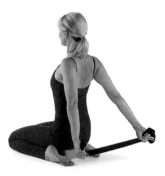

Fig. 3

Fig. 3

* Hold a yoga strap behind your back with your hands a comfortable distance apart.

* Move your shoulder blades down your back as you lift your chest and arms.

* Breathe for 5 to 10 evenly paced breaths.

* Exhale and release your arms.

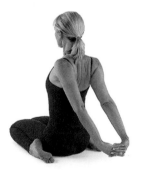

Fig. 4

Fig. 4: *Option for full pose*

* If you have the flexibility, sit on the floor between your knees, release the strap, and clasp your hands behind your back.

* Breathe for 5 to 10 evenly paced breaths.

* Exhale and release your hands and arms.

* Keeping your shoulders down, stretch your arms overhead, interlace your fingers, and turn your palms up. Lengthen the sides of your waist. Keep your lower-rib-to-hipbone connection (see Fig. 1).

* Exhale and release your hands and arms.

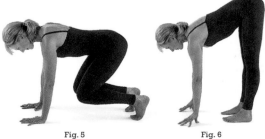

Fig. 5   Fig. 6

Figs. 5 and 6

* To stretch your legs, place your hands in front of you and turn your toes under.

* Lift your hips upward to straighten your knees; press your heels down. You will come to Standing Forward Bend (see p. 94).

* Inhale as you raise your upper body, keeping the spine long. Bring your arms out to the sides and then overhead. Exhale and release your arms to your sides.

COBRA POSE
BHUJANGASANA

Cobra Pose is a beginning back bend that teaches the body how to bend backward without working the already flexible areas of the spine, mainly the lower back. In Cobra Pose, the upper, less flexible area of the spine is gently extended, while the belly stays on the mat as support. This strengthens the upper back muscles and helps improve posture. If you practice this pose correctly, you should not feel compression in your lower back.

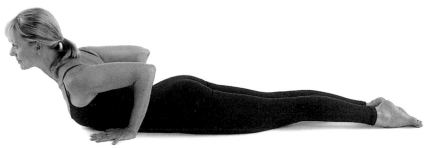

Fig. 1

Benefits

✳ Tones and strengthens the upper back

✳ Improves posture

✳ Helps relieve stiffness in upper spine

✳ Opens the chest for improved breathing

Things to remember

✳ *Keep pressing your pubic bone into the mat.*

✳ *Pull your abdominals away from the mat.*

✳ *Move your shoulder blades down your back.*

✳ *Keep your lower-rib-to-hipbone connection.*

✳ *Soften your eyes and focus internally.*

✳ *Lift from your upper back, not your head.*

✳ *Breathe.*

Tip

✳ This is a small lift from the floor with a strong movement of the shoulder blades downward.

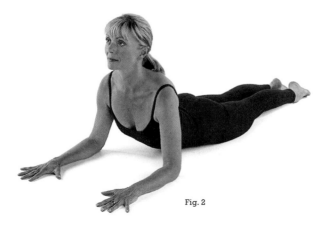

Fig. 2

Fig. 2

* Lie face down with your inner thighs connected.

* Place your elbows under your shoulders and your hands in line with your elbows. Press down through the length of your forearms and hands as you pull your shoulder blades down your back.

* Engage your abdominal muscles to support your back as you lift your chest forward.

* Press your pubic bone and legs into the mat. Keep your lower-rib-to-hipbone connection to avoid initiating this pose from your lower back.

* Lengthen your legs and press your feet into the mat.

* Breathe for 5 to 10 evenly paced breaths.

* Exhale and release your upper body to the mat. Feel the breath in the back of your body. Use Child's Pose (see p. 86) to release your back.

Fig. 3: *Incorrect position*

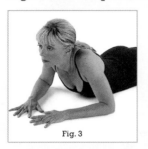

Fig. 3

* Do not allow your shoulders to press up to your ears.

* Keep your hands shoulder-width apart.

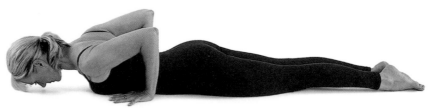

Fig. 4

Fig. 4: *Option for full pose*

* Place the heel of your hand in line with your lowest rib and your elbows above your wrists. Pull your shoulder blades down your back.

* Inhale, and as you exhale, press your pubic bone down, lengthen your legs, and lift your chest forward (see Fig. 1).

* Breathe for 5 to 10 long, evenly paced breaths.

* Exhale and release your body to the mat. Feel the breath in the back of your body. Use Child's Pose to release your back and rest.

LOCUST POSE
SALABHASANA

Locust Pose is a beginner's back bend that strengthens the entire back of the body from the upper spine to the lower legs. To avoid compressing your lower back, be sure to stabilize the back by engaging your abdominal muscles before lifting your legs. This pose is excellent for relieving tension in the shoulders. It also helps improve posture.

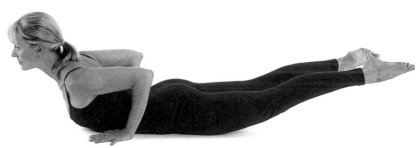

Fig. 1

Benefits

❋ Aids digestion

❋ Strengthens the entire back of the body

❋ Improves slumped posture

❋ Improves breathing

❋ Invigorates the mind, body, and spirit

Things to remember

❋ *Lift up from your middle spine, not your head and neck.*

❋ *Keep your pubic bone pressing into the mat to avoid compression in your lower spine.*

❋ *Lengthen more than you lift.*

❋ *Keep your shoulders down away from your ears.*

❋ *Breathe.*

Tip

❋ If lifting both legs causes strain, do this posture 2 to 4 times alternating right and left legs, holding for 3 to 5 evenly paced breaths.

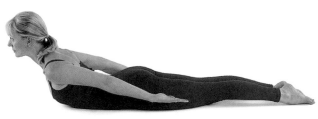
Fig. 2

Fig. 2

✻ Lie face down. Place your hands at your sides with your palms turned upward.

✻ Inhale, and as you exhale, stretch your fingers toward your toes to pull your shoulders down.

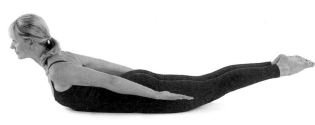
Fig. 3

Fig. 3

✻ Inhale, and as you exhale, press your pubic bone into the mat. Press your palms up as you lift your chest. Your head should follow the movement of the spine.

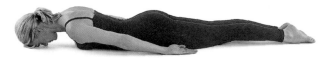
Fig. 4

Fig. 4: Modification

✻ Inhale, and as you exhale, with your upper body lifted, slowly lift your legs.

✻ Engage your abdominals as if lifting your belly away from the floor. Lengthen your body from your toes to the top of your head.

✻ Breathe for 5 to 10 long, evenly paced breaths.

✻ Exhale and release your body to the mat. Feel the breath in the back of your body. Use Child's Pose (see p. 86) to release your back and rest.

Option for full pose

✻ Place the heel of your hand in line with your lowest rib and your elbows above your wrists.

✻ Pull your shoulder blades down your back. Inhale, and as you exhale, press your pubic bone down, lengthen your legs, press your hands into the mat, and lift your chest forward.

✻ Slowly lift your legs and lengthen out through your body from head to toe (see Fig. 1).

✻ Breathe for 5 to 10 long, evenly paced breaths.

✻ Inhale, and as you exhale, slowly lower your body to the mat.

✻ Breath into the width of your back, then move back and rest in Child's Pose to release your back.

✻ Repeat 2 to 4 times.

BRIDGE POSE
SETU BANDHASANA

Bridge Pose strengthens the hips, buttocks, thighs, and lower and midback. It stretches the front of the thighs and the abdominal muscles. Variations of this pose are used in physical therapy as well as traditional fitness. As you lift, hold, and lower your body, yourattention should be focused on correct alignment and evenly paced breathing.

Things to remember

❋ *Never turn your head from side to side while in Bridge Pose.*

❋ *Your shoulder blades move down your back.*

❋ *Lengthen your neck; your chin should be an inch or so away from your collarbones.*

❋ *Keep your lower-rib-to-hipbone connection. Lift your chest without pressing your rib cage forward.*

❋ *Press down on your arms and heels to lift the spine evenly.*

❋ *Keep your shins vertical.*

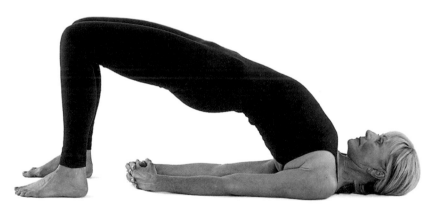

Fig. 1

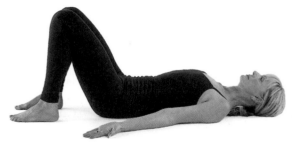

Fig. 2

Fig. 2

∗ Lie on your back, heels in line with your sit bones, arms at your sides, palms up, shoulders down, and neck long.

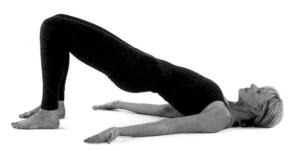

Fig. 3

Fig. 3

∗ Inhale, and as you exhale, press your heels down to lift your hips off the floor.

∗ The weight of your upper body should be distributed between your shoulder blades and the weight of your lower body over the four corners of your feet.

∗ Engage your inner thighs to keep them in a straight line from ankles to hips. Press your arms into the mat.

∗ Keep your lower-rib-to-hipbone connection.

∗ Point your tailbone toward your knees rather than your heels.

∗ Breathe for 5 to 10 evenly paced breaths.

∗ Exhale as you lower your upper body, rolling down one vertebra at a time from the top of your spine to your tailbone.

Option for full pose

∗ Inhale, and as you exhale, press your heels to lift your hips off the floor (see Fig. 3).

∗ Roll your weight to your left shoulder as you move your right shoulder blade down your back. Roll to the right and move your left shoulder blade down your back. Clasp your hands below you.

∗ Press the length of your arms into the mat as you continue to lift your chest and hips. Feel the weight of your body in your upper outer arms and heels (see Fig. 1).

∗ Breathe for 5 to 10 long, evenly paced breaths.

∗ Release your hands and widen your shoulder blades.

∗ Exhale as you lower your upper body, rolling down one vertebra at a time from the top of your spine through your tailbone.

BOW POSE
DHANURASANA

Bow Pose is one of the most recognized and invigorating of all yoga postures. It stretches the entire front of the body, the chest, the abdominals, and the pelvic region, which increases circulation for healthy organ function and better breathing. The back of the body is toned from head to heels for improved strength, flexibility, and posture. The following modification will teach you how to move into the full Bow Pose without compressing your lower back or straining your knees. Work carefully with the instructions to prepare your body and your breath.

Benefits

✻ Stretches and tones the abdominal organs and skin

✻ Relieves tension from the entire spinal column

✻ Improves posture

✻ Develops agility and poise

Things to remember

✻ *Keep your shoulder blades moving down your back.*

✻ *Maintain an even arch throughout your entire spinal column. If you feel compression in your lower back, lower your legs and focus more attention on the lower-rib-to-hipbone connection by engaging your abdominal muscles.*

Tip

✻ As you breathe, your body will naturally rock back and forth.

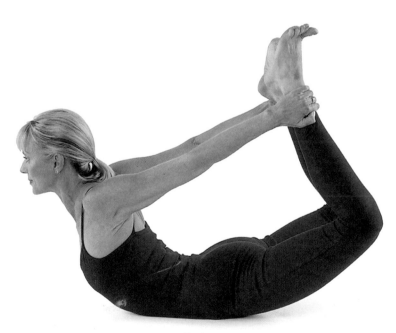

Fig. 1

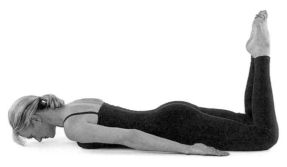

Fig. 2

Fig. 2

✳ Lie face down on the mat. Turn your palms up. Separate your inner thighs hip distance and bend your knees.

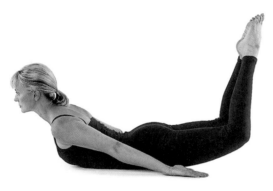

Fig. 3

Fig. 3

✳ Press your pubic bone into the mat and engage your hamstrings as you lift your knees off the mat.

✳ Inhale, and as you exhale, slide your hands back along the mat and roll your shoulders back as you lift your chest.

✳ Engage your abdominal muscles to protect your lower back.

✳ Breathe for 5 to 10 evenly paced breaths.

✳ Exhale and release. Breathe into the width and length of your back. Repeat two more times.

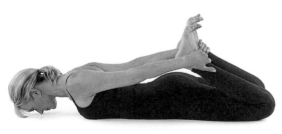

Fig. 4

Fig. 4: *Option for full pose*

✳ Hold your ankles with your palms facing each other. Lengthen the front of your thighs.

✳ Inhale to lengthen your body and exhale to engage your abdominal muscles.

✳ Inhale, and as you exhale, press your feet upward, lifting your chest from your upper back. Your head should follow the curve of the spine.

✳ Keep your hamstring and abdominal muscles engaged to protect your knees and support your lower back (see Fig. 1).

✳ Breathe for 5 to 10 long, evenly paced breaths.

✳ Exhale and release your body to the mat.

RECLINING LEG TWISTS

Some muscle groups wrap around the body in a diagonal plane. To receive maximum benefit when stretching and toning, a muscle must be addressed in the plane in which it lies. The following twists target the muscles of the chest, back, abdomen, and hips. When practiced consciously, twists are a safe and effective way to increase blood flow to the entire torso and are a beneficial aid to digestion and proper organ function.

Benefits

* Target muscle groups in the diagonal plane for maximum stretch and tone

* Aid digestion

* Feel great!

Things to remember

* *Use your breath to deepen your twist.*

* *Think of lengthening your spine as you twist.*

Tip

* Fig. 1 creates a slightly deeper chest stretch, while Fig. 3 is a deeper stretch through the lower back, hips, and waist.

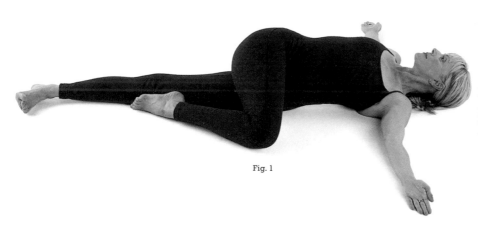

Fig. 1

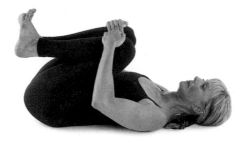

Fig. 2

Fig. 2

✳ Lie on your back with your knees pulled in to your chest.

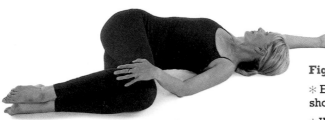

Fig. 3

Fig. 3

✳ Extend your arms straight out from your shoulders, palms up.

✳ With your exhalation, lower your knees to the right, all the way to the mat.

✳ Inhale, and as you exhale, turn your rib cage and your head away from your knees.

✳ For a deeper chest stretch, lengthen your right arm up toward your ear. Breathe deeply to deepen the stretch.

✳ Breathe for 5 to 10 long, evenly paced breaths.

✳ Exhale and bring your knees in to your chest as you return to center. Repeat on the opposite side.

Option for full pose

✳ Extend your arms straight out from your shoulders (see Fig. 1).

✳ Straighten your left leg and bring your right knee across your body to the left (see Fig. 1).

✳ Turn your rib cage and head to the right. Lengthen your body from your straight leg through the top of your head (see Fig. 1).

✳ Breathe for 5 to 10 long, evenly paced breaths.

✳ Exhale and return to center, knees to chest. Repeat on the other side.

BOAT POSE WITH WARM-UPS
NAVASANA WITH WARM-UPS

Toned abdominal muscles are essential for postural support and proper organ function. The following poses require your attention to proper contraction of the abdominal muscles and breath. Progress to the more difficult variations only when you can easily accomplish the modified versions.

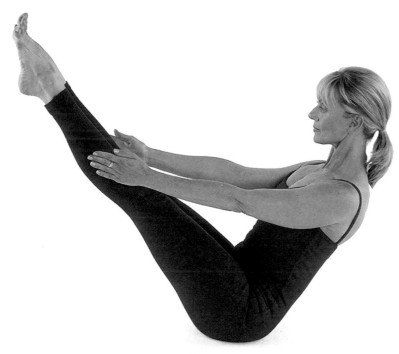

Fig. 1

Benefits

∗ Tones abdominal muscles and strengthens the back

∗ Improves function of liver and gall-bladder

Things to remember

∗ *Exhale to help engage your abdominal muscles.*

∗ *When lying down, do not allow your back to arch; keep your lower ribs on the mat.*

∗ *Progress to the seated variations only when you are comfortable in the reclining versions.*

∗ *Keep your shoulders down.*

∗ *Curl your chin in slightly toward your collarbones as you roll up.*

∗ *Straighten your knees only if you can control the position from your abdominal muscles.*

∗ *Breathe.*

Tip

∗ In order to keep your breath flowing and to maintain the abdominal contraction necessary to hold this pose, breathe into the back of your rib cage.

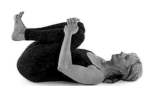

Fig. 2

Fig. 2

* Lie on your back with your knees pulled in to your chest.

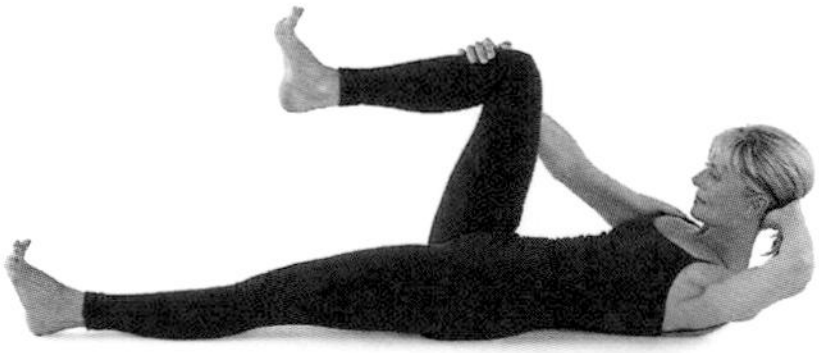

Fig. 3

* Exhale and stretch your left leg out along the mat.

* Inhale, and as you exhale, lengthen the back of your neck and roll up.

* Place your left hand behind your head for support and clasp your right hand around your right knee.

* Pull your abdominals in firmly as you stretch out through your straight leg.

* Keep your shoulder down and your neck long.

* Breathe for 5 to 10 long, evenly paced breaths.

* Exhale and roll down, releasing your head and knee. Bring your left leg in and repeat on the other side. Repeat each side 2 or 3 times.

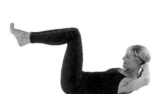

Fig. 3

Figs. 4 and 5

* With your knees pulled to your chest, place your hands behind your head.

* Inhale, and as you exhale, curl your upper body off the mat and move your knees over your hip sockets. Your shins should be horizontal.

* Hold and breathe for 5 to 10 evenly paced breaths, *or . . .*

* Inhale, and as you exhale, extend your legs straight and hold them at an angle that you can comfortably control. Stop if you feel a strain in your back.

* Breathe for 5 to 10 long, evenly paced breaths. Repeat 2 to 4 times.

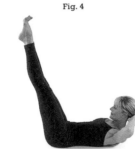

Fig. 4

Fig. 5

Fig. 6: *Option for full pose*

* Sit upright with your knees bent and your feet in front of you. Hold the backs of your calves and lean back. Lift your feet so that your shins are horizontal to the floor.

* When you have your balance, stretch your fingers to your toes. Engage your deep, lower abdominal muscles from your pubic bone to your hipbones.

* When you can maintain balance and stability though your abdomen, extend and straighten your legs (see Fig. 1).

* Breathe for 5 to 10 evenly paced breaths.

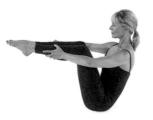

Fig. 6

SAGE TWIST
BHARADVAJASANA

Twists are an essential element in a balanced yoga practice. They directly affect the spine and the function of the abdominal organs. It is important to remember to lengthen your spine and continue lengthening as you twist. Think of gently twisting your spine from its base upward through the crown of your head. Always inhale to lengthen and exhale to twist.

Benefits

* Stimulates and tones abdominal organs

* Aids digestion

* Releases spinal tension

* Warms and invigorates

Things to remember

* *Keep your shoulders down and your chest lifted.*

* *Lift your chest as if lifting your entire spine up from its base.*

* *Lead the twist from your lower belly; your shoulders and head just follow the movement.*

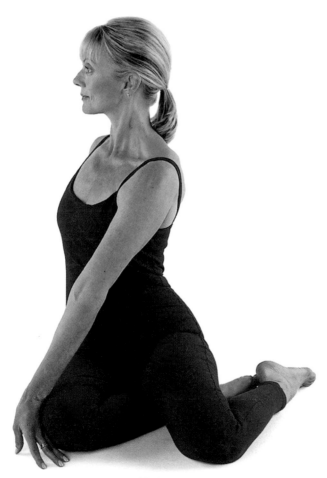

Fig. 1

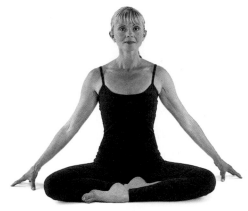

Fig. 2

Fig. 2

* Sit in a simple cross-legged position. Place your fingertips on the floor behind you. Inhale and lengthen your spine.

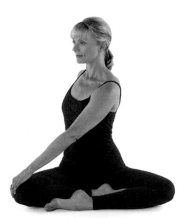

Fig. 3

Fig. 3

* With your exhalation, begin to twist to the right. Inhale to lengthen and exhale to twist.

* Breathe for 5 to 10 long, evenly paced breaths.

* Come back to center and change sides, twisting to the left.

* Breathe for 5 to 10 long, evenly paced breaths.

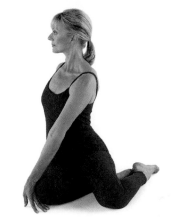

Fig. 4

Fig. 4: *Option for full pose*

* Sit with your legs extended in front of you. Pull the flesh out from underneath your buttocks and sit upright on your pelvis.

* Point your toes and sweep your feet to the left.

* Inhale, lengthen your spine, exhale, and twist to your right. With each inhalation, lengthen your spine, and with each exhalation, twist a little deeper.

* Breathe for 5 to 10 evenly paced breaths.

* Exhale and release. Repeat on the opposite side.

SINGLE-LEG SEATED TWIST
MARICHYASANA III

This is a seated lateral twist. In this pose, one side of the abdomen is compressed while the other is stretched. The effect of this posture on the internal organs is similar to that of wringing out a sponge. When compressed, the organs release toxins. When the compression is released, they are able to absorb more oxygen and fresh nutrients. This pose is particularly effective to detoxify and invigorate the liver, spleen, and intestines.

Benefits

* Tones abdominal muscles

* Relieves stiffness in the hips, back, and spine

Things to remember

* *If your lower back is rounded when seated on the floor, sit on a blanket.*

* *Move with your breath.*

* *Lengthen as much as you twist.*

* *Turn from your torso; your shoulders and head follow.*

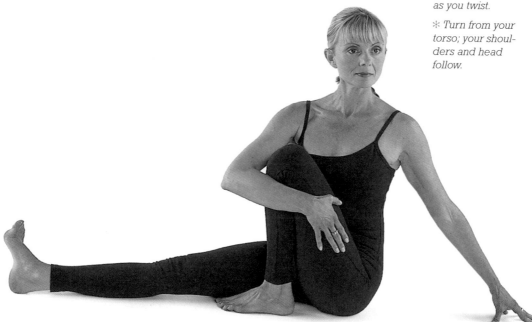

Fig. 1

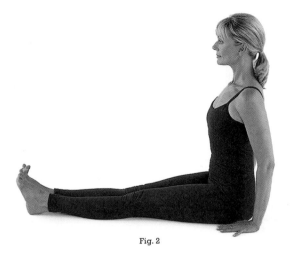

Fig. 2

Fig. 2

❊ Begin in Staff Pose (see p. 134). Pull your sit bones back, extend your legs, and lengthen your spine.

❊ If your lower back is rounded, sit on a firmly folded blanket to raise your hips slightly.

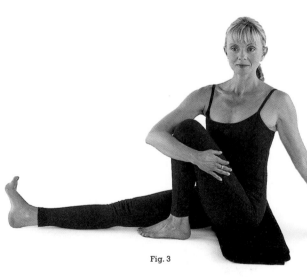

Fig. 3

Fig. 3

❊ Bend your right knee and place your right heel in line with your right outer hip.

❊ Keep your left leg fully extended and flex your left foot, keeping your heel on the mat.

❊ Place your left arm across your right knee, twisting toward your bent knee.

❊ Inhale to lengthen your spine and exhale to twist. With each inhalation, lengthen your spine, and with each exhalation, twist a little deeper. Twist from your waist and spiral upward through your neck.

❊ Keep the axis of your spine straight from your tailbone through the top of your head.

❊ Breathe for 5 to 10 long, evenly paced breaths.

❊ Exhale and release, turning back to center. Repeat on the other side.

Option for full pose

❊ When you have attained flexibility in your hips and strength through your torso, remove the blanket (see Fig. 1).

SINGLE-LEG SEATED FORWARD BEND

JANUSIRSASANA

It is always tempting to try to push ahead before the body is ready to do so. It is particularly important in the seated forward bends that you use enough support (blankets and straps) and never force yourself to move more deeply than is comfortable for your body. When this pose is practiced consciously, it's excellent for relieving tension in the back and hips. It has a strong toning effect upon the liver, spleen, and kidneys. Because this is an asymmetrical pose, you need to pay attention to the position of the pelvis, keeping the hipbones in the same plane.

Benefits

* Tones and detoxifies the internal organs

* Helps relieve back stiffness

Things to remember

* *Don't force your body too deeply into the stretch.*

* *Move with your breath.*

* *Keep your shoulder blades moving down your back.*

* *Lengthen your spine.*

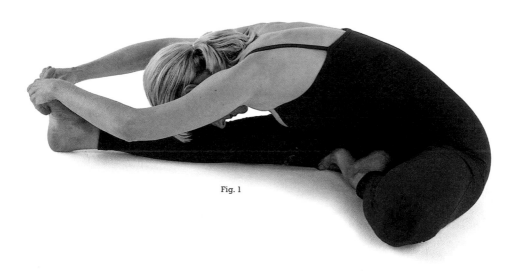

Fig. 1

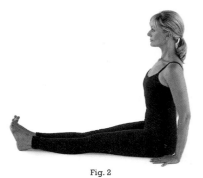

Fig. 2

Fig. 2

* Begin in Staff Pose (see p. 134). Pull your sit bones back, extend your legs straight, and lengthen your spine.

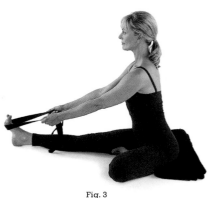

Fig. 3

Fig. 3

* Bend your right knee and place the sole of your right foot high on your inner left thigh.

* Lower your right knee to the mat.

* Place a strap around the ball of your left foot, holding it with both hands. If your lower back is rounded, sit on a folded blanket to raise your hips slightly.

* Lengthen your spine and keep your shoulder blades down and your abdominals engaged.

* Breathe for 5 to 10 long, evenly paced breaths.

* Exhale and release, change legs, and repeat on the other side.

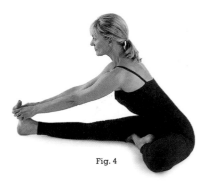

Fig. 4

Fig. 4: *Option for full pose*

* If you feel you have attained flexibility, release the strap and remove the blanket. Inhale and lengthen your spine; then exhale and reach forward to hold the inner and outer left foot.

* Keep your shoulder blades moving down your back and your abdominals engaged.

* As you hold your foot, lift your chest. Continue breathing and lengthening your spine as you stretch your inner right thigh and the back of your left leg.

* As you increase your flexibility, fold forward over your leg without collapsing (see Fig. 1).

* Continue to lengthen your spine, engage your abdominals, and breathe.

* Breathe for 5 to 10 evenly paced breaths.

* Inhale as you come up. Change legs and repeat on the other side.

STAFF POSE
DANDASANA

This pose is deceiving. It looks simple, but it requires the use of the abdominal, back, and thigh muscles and focused concentration. Be conscious of the interaction between the mind and body. As you lose your awareness of your breath, you will notice that your mind has wandered and your body has lost the posture. This is a great place to challenge the mind-body connection and safely strengthen many major muscle groups.

Benefits

* Teaches integration of mind and body

* Teaches awareness of moving in two directions simultaneously

* Tones the entire body

* Tones the waist

* Helps to balance the pelvis after asymmetrical seated forward bends

Things to remember

* *Sit upright on your pelvis.*

* *Reach though your heels; flex your feet and ankles.*

* *Keep your heels on the mat.*

* *Strongly move your legs and shoulders down and your spine up.*

* *Remain conscious of your breath.*

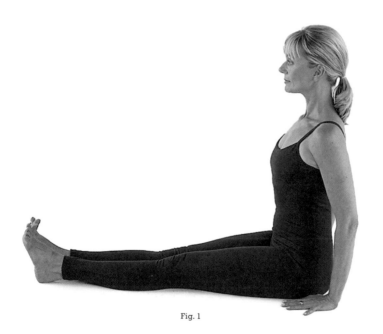

Fig. 1

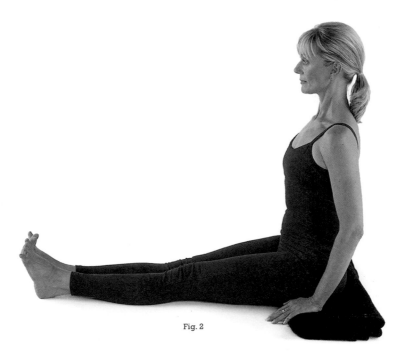

Fig. 2

Fig. 2

✳ Sit with straight legs. Pull the flesh out from underneath your buttocks and sit upright on your sit bones.

✳ Sitting on a blanket will help keep your pelvis in correct alignment.

✳ Place your arms beside you, hands on the blanket.

✳ Flex your feet and extend out through your heels, pulling your toes back toward you.

✳ Keep the backs of your thighs pressed to the floor. Lengthen your spine upward though the top of your head, shoulders down.

✳ Breathe for 5 to 10 long, evenly paced breaths.

SEATED FORWARD BEND
PASCHIMOTTANASANA

Seated Forward Bend is powerfully relaxing. It stretches the spine but also literally folds the body in half, which turns our awareness inward. This is a wonderful pose to finish up a yoga practice or to help induce restful sleep. Remember, it is the integrity that you bring to every pose that is important, not how far you go.

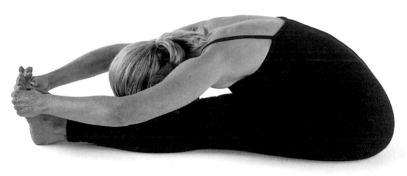

Fig. 1

Benefits

* Tones and massages abdominal organs and pelvic region

* Aids digestion

* Stimulates kidneys

* Soothes the nervous system

* Calms the mind

Things to remember

* *Sit upright; do not allow your lower back to round or your chest to slump even as you fold forward.*

* *Keep your legs straight, feet and ankles flexed.*

* *Use enough strap to feel the stretch in the back of your legs, not your lower back.*

* *Sit on a blanket if needed to keep your pelvis in an upright position.*

* *Feel your spine moving upward, your legs pressing downward.*

* *Keep your shoulders down and arms straight.*

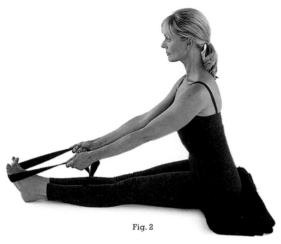

Fig. 2

Fig. 2

* From Staff Pose (see p. 134), place a strap around your feet. Press into the strap with the balls of your feet, spreading your toes.

* Keep your arms straight and shoulders down. Lift into your chest.

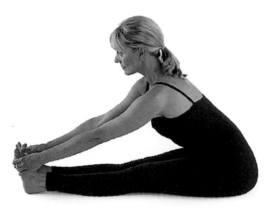

Fig. 3

Fig. 3: *Option for full pose*

* Remove the strap and hold the outsides of your feet.

* Place your thumbs on the knuckles of your big toes and press forward.

* Lift into your chest.

* Fold forward from your hips, not your lower back.

* Breathe for 5 to 10 evenly paced breaths.

* Inhale as you come up.

CORPSE POSE
SAVASANA

As you know, yoga has a powerful effect upon the nervous system. All variations of yoga practices have one thing in common: Relaxation at the end of the poses. This is essential to achieving a quality of mind and body that is balanced and clear. During relaxation, your body should be in a reclined position. The traditional relaxation posture is done flat on the floor. You may find that your body needs more support. Included are some suggestions for complete relaxation. If you are overheated or in a drafty space, make sure that you cover up so as not to get chilled.

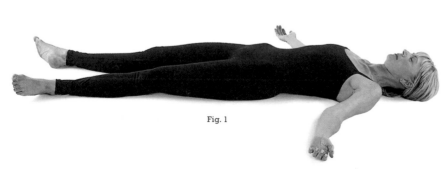

Fig. 1

Benefits

* Brings the nervous system to neutral after practice

* Trains the mind to observe the body in complete stillness

Thing to remember

* *Always take time to practice this pose and position so that your body feels perfectly balanced right to left and top to bottom. Then, let go.*

Tip

* If you find it difficult to lie still, give your mind something to focus on. Begin at your toes. Relax them with an exhalation. Move up your feet, relaxing your arches; the tops of your feet; your ankles, shins, and thighs. Relax your abdomen and feel your lower back release as if softening into the floor. Continue up your body through your spine, shoulders, arms, and fingers. Relax the muscles around your mouth, eyes, forehead, and temples. Now release your jaw and allow your throat to open so that your breath flows easily.

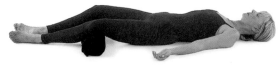

Fig. 2

Fig. 2: Variation 1

⁎ Place a rolled blanket under your knees for support.

⁎ Lie flat on your back.

⁎ Separate your knees a comfortable distance. Move your shoulder blades down your back and widen them.

⁎ Turn your palms up. Lengthen your neck and place the center of your head on the mat.

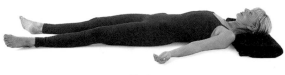

Fig. 3

Fig. 3: Variation 2

⁎ Place a thinly folded blanket under your head and neck to give enough support so that your chin doesn't tip upward. The blanket should just touch the top of your shoulders.

⁎ Turn your palms up. Lengthen your neck and place the center of your head on the mat.

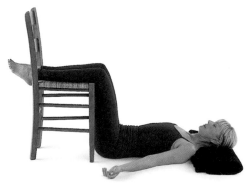

Fig. 4

Fig. 4: Variation 3

⁎ Place a chair under your lower legs. The chair should come to the back of your knees.

⁎ Place a thinly folded blanket under your head and neck. The blanket should just touch the top of your shoulders.

⁎ Lengthen your neck and place the center of your head on the mat. Turn your palms up.

Option for full pose

⁎ Lie flat on your back and take the time to position yourself. Your body should be balanced, right to left (see Fig. 1).

⁎ Position your shoulder blades evenly wide and down your back. Your ribcage should be evenly placed, right to left on the mat.

⁎ Separate your legs evenly and make sure your head is in the center of the mat (see Fig. 1).

⁎ Once you have balanced yourself, take a few long, slow, deep, evenly paced breaths. Allow your body to sink into the mat.

INDEX

Complement your collection with yoga programs on DVD and video!

Great for anyone ready to create a balanced, healthy lifestyle!

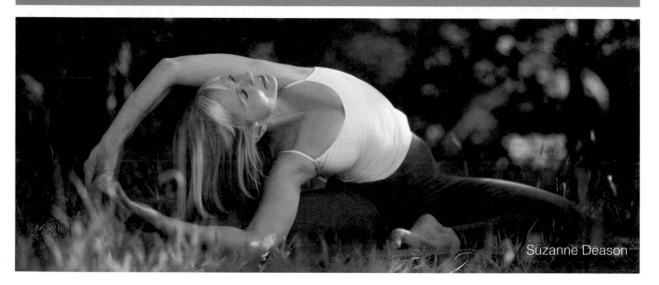

Suzanne Deason

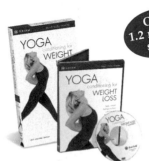

Over 1.2 million sold!

Yoga Conditioning for Weight Loss VHS *Award winner!*

A unique, ground-breaking workout to restore and maintain your ideal weight. Accommodates all levels of fitness by simultaneously demonstrating four levels of modification. As your energy and stamina increase, you progress to the next level. A healthful, long-term weight loss plan to balance the mind, body and spirit. With Suzanne Deason. *60 minutes.*

Yoga Conditioning for Weight Loss DVD *Award winner!*

The deluxe DVD edition includes the complete three-part, multi-level workout, three individual fitness level variations, angle feature that allows you to change your workout level during the program, fully chaptered workout to let you to navigate the parts of the workout, additional on-screen instruction with our exclusive Pose Guide feature, in-depth interview with Suzanne Deason, and booklet with nutrition and weight management tips. *4 hours 20 minutes.*

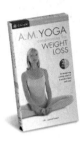
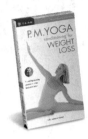
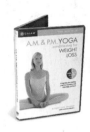

A.M. Yoga Conditioning for Weight Loss VHS

A short, morning yoga practice to get in touch with the needs of the body and inspire the connection of body, mind and spirit throughout the day. The practice begins with seated breathing awareness to gently center yourself and eases you into a series of modified standing and seated postures paying special attention on breathing to promote circulation. With Suzanne Deason. *30 minutes.*

P.M. Yoga Conditioning for Weight Loss VHS

A short, evening yoga practice to restore the connection of the body, mind and spirit at the end of the day and remind us how our choices affect the way we look and feel. The practice begins with standing breathing awareness to ground you in the present and eases you into a sequence of modified postures to release tension, calm nerves and enhance circulation. With Suzanne Deason. *30 minutes.*

A.M./P.M. Yoga Conditioning for Weight Loss DVD

The deluxe DVD edition includes the modified morning and evening yoga practices, bonus yoga practice to explore the full postures with breathing and an in-depth interview with Suzanne Deason. *1 hour 30 minutes.*

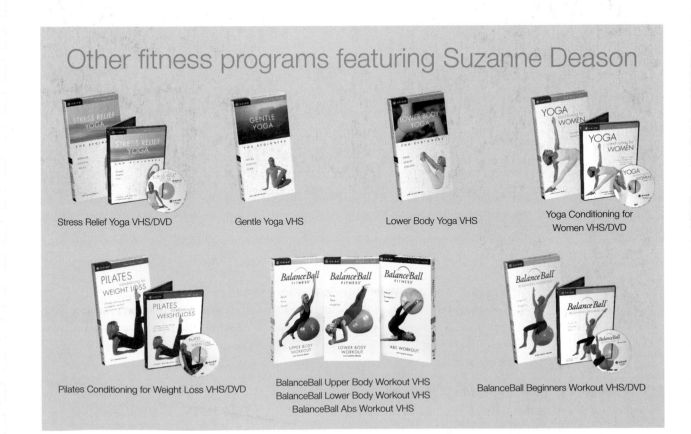
TO ORDER 800.254.8464 | www.gaiam.com

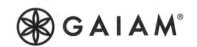

A LIFESTYLE COMPANY
for
HEALTH AND SUSTAINABILITY

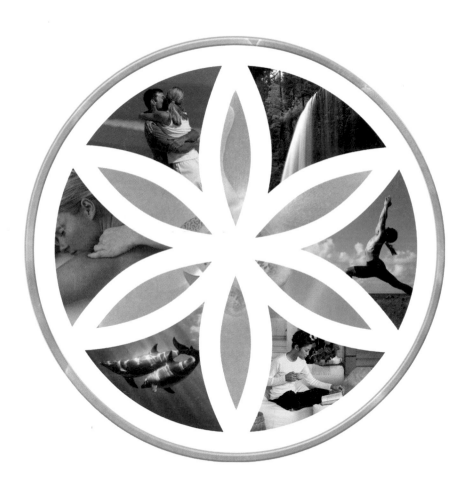

GAIAM®

www.gaiam.com
800.254.8464